NUTRITION AND DIET RESEARCH PROGRESS

MALNUTRITION

PREVALENCE, RISK FACTORS AND OUTCOMES

NUTRITION AND DIET RESEARCH PROGRESS

Additional books and e-books in this series can be found on Nova's website under the Series tab.

NUTRITION AND DIET RESEARCH PROGRESS

MALNUTRITION

PREVALENCE, RISK FACTORS AND OUTCOMES

AZIZUR RAHMAN
EDITOR

nova
Medicine & Health
New York

Library of Congress Cataloging-in-Publication Data

Names: Rahman, Azizur (Associate Professor in Mathematics and Statistics), editor.
Title: Malnutrition : prevalence, risk factors and outcomes / [edited by] Azizur Rahman.
Description: Hauppauge : Nova Science Publishers, [2020] | Series: Prevalence, risk factors and outcomes | Includes bibliographical references and index. |
Identifiers: LCCN 2020008196 (print) | LCCN 2020008197 (ebook) | ISBN 9781536175974 (hardcover) | ISBN 9781536175981 (adobe pdf)
Subjects: LCSH: Malnutrition--Epidemiology. | Malnutrition--Risk factors.
Classification: LCC RA645.N87 M362 2020 (print) | LCC RA645.N87 (ebook) | DDC 614.5/939--dc23
LC record available at https://lccn.loc.gov/2020008196
LC ebook record available at https://lccn.loc.gov/2020008197

Published by Nova Science Publishers, Inc. † New York

To my parents and family

CONTENTS

PREFACE

This book composes a wide range of contemporary research from leading international experts of the malnutrition field. It covers socioeconomic, demographic, clinical, and environmental and policy related malnutrition topics and explores the theme of the prevalence, risk factors and outcomes of malnutrition lifecycle and burden of the 21st century's world.

Malnutrition affects the future productivity of a society and it is an associated cause in about half of all deaths occurring among children in developing countries with severe malnutrition associated with 1 to 2 million preventable child deaths each year. According to the UNICEF, recent global estimates indicate that nearly 60 million children have a moderate form of malnutrition, and 13 million have a severe form of malnutrition. Additionally, nutritional status assessment serves as a means for evaluating the health condition and survival of children, and also provides indirect measurements of a range of significant indicators in public health, socioeconomic developments and the quality of life of a population. It is necessary to highlight the widespread malnutrition issues – especially among the children and mother in many countries, risk factors and policy implications at national, regional and international levels since developed worlds are assisting on such issues through various aid programs. Therefore, comprehensive research on malnutrition is significant and an important international interest. As a result this book brings together seven state-of-the-arts research chapters on significant topics which are rigorously peer reviewed.

The first chapter focuses on the aging related malnutrition and poor quality of life due to its chronicity, community, and emotional viewpoints. Increase in lifespan, demographic modification demands for a foremost determination to confirm the quality of life in our geriatric population. Since nutrition is an important part for the elderly that affects their immunity and working ability, therefore, it warrants attention in elderly care. Malnutrition is common in the older age (60% prevalence rate) and the depression is one of the correctable risk factors. There are other risk factors such as frailty, age, unnecessary polypharmacy, health decline in general, difficulty in eating/swallowing, and socializing. Previous research has shown a bidirectional link between depression and nutritional status of people. Depression and nutrition independently also contribute to decreased health-related quality of life (HR-QOL) among the elderly. Malnutrition can be increased by several factors such as dependency on others for daily routine, being alone, chronic sickness, and it forces morbidness, death, and poor quality of life.

The second chapter presents a cross-sectional research to assess the prevalence of malnutrition among rural primary school children utilizing new internationally accepted age and sex specific cut offs of body mass index (BMI). The study was conducted among 822 rural primary school children of Jangipara Block of Hooghly District, West Bengal, India. A total of 812 children (431 girls; 381 boys) aged from 6 to 10 years were eligible for the research. Results indicated that girls were thinner than boys. In contrast, boys were prone to be overweight and obese. All regional studies (including the present) had reported very high prevalence rate of overall thinness according to World Health Organization. Most of the international and national studies had observed a lower rate of overall thinness than our study. In conclusion, the present study clearly indicated that half of the studied girls (50.6%) were undernourished and more boys were overweight and obese. Surveillance of present nutritional schemes and state specific appropriate and immediate new nutritional interventions are required to ameliorate the problem of malnutrition.

The third chapter presents results of the prevalence and the key determinants of acute malnutrition in rural children in Bangladesh. This study used nationally representative data from the 2014 Bangladesh Demographic Health and Survey (BDHS). Chi-square test was performed to investigate the association between outcome variables and selected covariates. Multinomial logistic regression was used to identify factors associated with acute malnutrition. Findings reveal that all the selected factors in this study were significant at (p-value <0.10) in Chi-square test. The overall estimated prevalence rates of acute malnutrition in rural Bangladeshi children was 16.7%; among them 12.2% were moderately wasted ($-3.0 \leq$ Z-score < -2.0) and 4.5% severely wasted (Z-score<-3.0). In the multinomial regression, being male children, smaller than average size at birth, low maternal BMI ($\leq$18.50 kg/m^2), short maternal height (<145cm) and poor index household were found to be significant determinants for acute malnutrition among children under five in rural Bangladesh. Finally, this chapter shows how understanding of those factors might enable to design and targeting any preventive-intervention programs or policies towards stopping and improving the child acute malnutrition in the rapidly growing developing country.

The fourth chapter is a methodologically advanced research addressing issues related to the governments and policy makers focus more on public health indicators at disaggregated level administrative units. The World Bank small area estimation (SAE) method known as ELL method has been widely used for estimating poverty and child malnutrition at micro-level administrative units for many developing countries using continuous response variables like household expenditure and children height-for-age Z-score (HAZ). However, health indicators like diarrhoea prevalence are based on categorical attributes and hence the ELL method cannot be implemented directly. The idea of ELL approach can be implemented after developing a generalized linear mixed model for the categorical response variable. An ELL type SAE approach has been proposed for binary response variable and evaluated through simulation studies and an empirical study using children HAZ data extracted from Bangladesh Demographic and Health Survey 2011 and the 5% of 2011 Census data.

District level estimates of stunting (HAZ < -2.00) and severe stunting (HAZ < -3.00) are calculated considering both continuous and binary response variables for examining the performance of the proposed SAE method. Findings of both simulation and empirical studies reveal feasibility of the SAE method for binary response variable.

Additionally, the fifth chapter presents Malnutrition and Age-Specific Child Mortality Burden in India as Child survival is one of the prominent indicators of child health. Over one-third of all child deaths are linked to malnutrition. To examine the significance of socio- economic factors and intergenerational transmission factors associated with age specific mortality by using National Family Health Survey Data (NFHS-3), this research uses the Cox proportional hazard models and life table techniques are used to determine the statistical significance of the variables used in the study. The results shows that factors such as gender, birth order, birth interval, birth size have substantial effects on mortality. Girls of higher birth order survive more during the first month than boys and reversal is true where later born boys have survival advantage after the first month up to five years. Intergenerational transmission variables like mother height, weight, age of mother at first birth, diet patterns, and health seeking behaviour are highly associated with all age specific mortality. There exists a strong association of domestic violence variable with neonatal mortality. Among the environmental features, the interaction term of open defecation with religion supports the findings from earlier studies that Muslim children have better survival advantage than their Hindu counterparts. This is due to the fact that open defecation is more in Hindu concentrated regions of rural areas and consequently the Hazard ratios for Muslims are lower when compared with Hindus. Short-term policies such as guidance and support for creating awareness on antenatal check-ups, institutional deliveries, longer birth intervals, shorter birth orders will help to curb the mortality of children.

Chapter six endeavours to examine the factors associated with underweight in rural Bangladeshi children. Nationally representative data from The Bangladesh Demographic and Health Survey (BDHS) 2014 data set was used for the study. A total of 4881 under-five year's aged children from rural areas were included in this study. An estimated of 35.1% of children aged under five years were underweight, whereas 26.1% moderately and 9% were severely underweight. Chi-square test was performed to examine the association between weight-for-age status and the selected covariates. Multinomial logistic regression was used to identify the associated factors with childhood underweight. Geographic division, child age, size at birth, fever and diarrhoea episode, mother's age at first birth, maternal BMI (kg/m^2), father's education, wealth index, toilet facilities and number of under-5 children were significantly associated with different form of underweight. As malnutrition is an amendable disease, therefore, it is important and implements with enough interventions to prevent, diagnose and treat malnutrition. The study also suggested significant recommendations to health policymakers that a national level perspective is necessary while designing the health policies and programs for children in rural Bangladesh.

The last chapter uses the big data analysis techniques to mitigate child malnutrition in developing countries. Geographical conditions, poverty index, education level, food habits, cultural traditions may play significant role when deciding malnutrition. Further, country to country impact of these factors may vary. Considering current state of the art there is no such study investigate means of child malnutrition (age under 5 years) in Sri Lankan context. So, the principal objective of this chapter is to establish a knowledge rich environment for related parties to make decisions to reduce child malnutrition condition in a developing country context (e.g. Sri Lanka) by considering rule based data mining techniques. Experimental results show that the education of the parents, access for media for the knowledge, proper understanding of family planning are crucial factors from preventing children falling into malnutrition condition. Findings also reveal that "Tamil" ethnicity shows higher probability to malnourished due to food consumption pattern. Furthermore, lack of nutrition during pregnancy impacts child health and malnutrition condition.

ACKNOWLEDGMENTS

The editor would like to take this opportunity to thank the authors, reviewers and the publishing team members for their excellent work and cooperation. Each manuscript was anonymously peer reviewed by at least two reviewers, who gave review feedback, objective and/or helpful revision comments to the authors where necessary. So, the outcome has made this volume of a very high quality. As it covers the key issues in malnutrition, this timely volume will be significant resources for the postgraduate to expert researchers, practitioners and policymakers.

Azizur Rahman
Wagga Wagga, New South Wales, Australia
December, 2019

In: Malnutrition
Editor: Azizur Rahman
ISBN: 978-1-53617-597-4

Chapter 1

MALNUTRITION: REVIEW OF PREVALENCE, RISK FACTORS AND OUTCOMES IN GERIATRIC POPULATION

***Manjula Suri*[1,*] *and Suneel Kumar*[2]**
[1]Department of Physiology and Promotive Health,
Institute of Home Economics, University of Delhi, New Delhi, India
[2]Department of Biomedical Engineering, Rutgers,
The State University of New Jersey, Piscataway, NJ, US

ABSTRACT

Aging leads to poor quality of life due to its chronicity, community, and emotional viewpoints. An increase in lifespan, demographic modification demands for a foremost determination to confirm the quality of life in our geriatric population. Since nutrition is an important part of the elderly that affects their immunity and working ability, therefore, it warrants attention in elderly care. Although, it is a multidimensional perception in the elderly with related emotional/psychological and physical elements. Malnutrition can be increased by several factors such as dependency on others for daily routine, being alone, chronic sickness, and it forces morbidness, death, and poor quality of life. Malnutrition is

* Corresponding Author's Email: mnjlsuri@gmail.com.

common in the older age (60% prevalence rate) and depression is one of the correctable risk factors. There are other risk factors such as frailty, age, unnecessary polypharmacy, health decline in general, difficulty in eating/swallowing, and socializing. Previous research has shown a bidirectional link between depression and the nutritional status of people. Depression and nutrition independently also contribute to decreased health-related quality of life (HR-QOL) among the elderly in the nutrition-depression-HR-QOL triad. Therefore, HR-QOL should not only be used to detect and treat depression among the elderly but also examine their nutrition status. A pilot study conducted by our gerontology students found a high frequency of malnutrition, pain, depression-related symptoms, and anxiety amongst the elderly urban population which was like that found in the rural population. Previous researchers have shown other risk factors like polypharmacy (use of multiple medicines concurrently) can cause a 2-fold more risk of malnutrition. Pathological risk factors causing inadvertent bodyweight loss that can also raise the risk of malnutrition, therefore, it is important to prevent or treat secondary illness in the elderly. Aging induces the decrement in functional and physiological activities such as senses (taste, smell, eyesight, etc.), dental health, which may also affect nutrient intake in these people. Malnutrition risk is also associated with a person's economic and social involvement. Socioeconomic factors include social isolation, poverty, and lack of independence which is connected to poor or no appetite. A significant association was also observed between malnutrition and those who do not have a pension. The identification of these factors in senior citizens is critically expanding an integrated malnutrition assessment tool that considers all risk factors. To conclude, it is important that health policymakers should consider nutritional perspective while formulating the health policies for the geriatric population. Since malnutrition is an amendable factor, it is important to develop and implement adequate interventions to prevent, diagnose, and treat malnutrition. Nutrition counsel services should also be made available to the elderly population for their better quality of life.

1. Introduction

The geriatric population is increasing worldwide and this growth will increase the global burden on healthcare services. Inadequate diet is common in the elderly and is due to numerous physiologic and socioeconomic factors. Therefore, health care workers and policymakers must be aware of the prevalence, risk factors, and outcomes of malnutrition among the elderly. Nutrition is an important contributing factor to the health and wellbeing of the elderly. Malnutrition is defined as a condition of the disproportion of protein, energy, and other nutrients that can negatively affect physical function, body composition, and related clinical outcomes (Elia 2000; Rahman and Chowdhury 2007; Rahman and Biswas 2009). Malnutrition includes both under and over-nutrition. Malnourished elderly will need more services such as health, social, and rehabilitation. Therefore, early diagnosis and treatment are essential for the prevention of malnutrition in the elderly (Kansal et al. 2016).

The geriatric population's nutritional requirements are diverse. Deficiencies in vitamins, minerals and a number of other nutrients/micronutrients are relatively common and can impact the quality of life (Rahman and Harding 2013; Rahman and Sapkota 2014; Leslie and Hankey 2015). The aging itself, however, neither leads to malabsorption or to malnutrition but may cause atrophic gastritis in the elderly. Researchers have reported that malnutrition is an independent risk factor for worse prognosis and increased morbidity as well as mortality (Pirlich and Lochs 2001; Rahman and Hakim 2016). Various physiological, pathological, socioeconomic, behavioral and food accessibility risk factors may contribute to the development of malnutrition in the elderly e.g., dental disorders, depression, loneliness, cognitive decline, financial problems, diarrheal diseases, etc. (Rahman and Harding 2011).

In general, malnutrition values are derived from younger adults and may not necessarily be suitable for elderly persons (Pirlich and Lochs 2001; Hasan et al. 2016; Hakim and Rahman 2016). The nutritional status of the elderly can be evaluated by various tools e.g., the body mass index, the Mini Nutritional Assessment Short Form (MNA-SF). The MNA-SF is a standardized questionnaire used for detecting malnutrition and screening version, the MNA-SF has good diagnostic accuracy. The MNA-SF will determine deficiency disease as well as "at risk of malnutrition" status (Rubenstein et al. 2001). The nutritional status of the elderly can be improved by methods such as a balanced oral diet, nutritional supplementation or enteral nutrition. Protein-energy deficiency disease has an impact on the elderly, their families, communities as well as the healthcare system. Health education and community awareness about malnutrition are important in detecting and managing this geriatric syndrome.

Various health outcomes of malnutrition in the elderly are poor physical health, poor mental health, poor bone health, and poor morbidity as well as mortality rate (Rahman et al. 2016). These outcomes may present as frailty, depression, pain, osteoporosis, delayed wound healing, etc. Therefore, treatment with special emphasis on psychosocial factors is the need of the hour in this frail population. As some studies revealed that malnutrition is associated with depressive symptoms, therefore, emotional and social well-being are the key factors for maintaining a healthy environment for the elderly (Mokhber et al. 2011; Hickson 2006). Researchers have shown that nutritional supplements improve depression in the elderly (Al-Rasheed et al. 2018). So, co-morbidity of malnutrition and depression must make us vigilant enough to refer our elderly patients to nutritionists to be fully worked up according to their nutritional status and their socioeconomic conditions (Mokhber et al. 2011). Another outcome of malnutrition is anxiety. Certain dietary factors may help in reducing anxiety e.g., a balanced diet, proper hydration and reducing or avoiding alcohol and caffeine (Naidoo 2016). The gut-brain axis is another important factor in the development of anxiety as well as depression. Therefore, researchers are examining the effect of probiotics in the treatment of malnutrition, depression, and anxiety (Messaoudi et al. 2011). Pain also interferes with food intake and may lead to weight loss, and malnutrition (Silva et al. 2013). Pain intensities are higher in undernourished elderly. Other serious outcomes of malnutrition are increased morbidity and mortality in general and lower cognitive state, osteoporosis, falls, fractures, in particular. To summarize, interactions between nutrition and the aging process are a challenging field of research and nutrition-based management is useful in preventing deficiency diseases in the geriatric population.

2. Prevalence of Malnutrition in the Elderly

Malnutrition is commonly observed in the geriatric population worldwide (Elia 2000). Malnutrition is a major public health concern as it affects every third person globally according to the 2016 Global Nutrition Report (Table 1). A retrospective pooled analysis from twelve countries has shown that the prevalence of deficiency disease was approximately twenty-three percent in the elderly. Prevalence of malnutrition was 50.5% in rehabilitation, 38.7% in hospital, 13.8% in nursing homes, and 5.8% in community settings (Kaiser et al. 2010).

Malnutrition prevalence in Europe and North American is 1-15% in non-institutionalized elderly. Malnutrition was found to be higher in geriatric care facilities (25–60%) and in hospitals (35–65%) (Gil-Montoya et al. 2013). The population between 2010 and 2050 will show growth from 11.5% to 21.0% worldwide and from 9.0% to 19.0% in the developed countries in the age group of> 80 years (World Population Prospects 2019). This will cause an increased prevalence of malnutrition in the geriatric population (Zeanandin et al. 2012). The prevalence of deficiency disease varies in several population subgroups and it is reported to be higher in elderly with deteriorating health, functional status, dependency, and disability. Besides prevalent malnutrition, the risk of developing malnutrition is also higher in the elderly (Kaiser et al. 2010b; Cereda 2012). Previously, it has been reported that about 27% of the Spanish elderly were at high risk of malnutrition (Julio et al. 2018). Another study was done in Turkey also showed that the proportion of elderly at risk of malnutrition was found to be 18.6% using MNA scores (Nazan and Buket 2018). A study conducted in Sweden and stated that people >80 years of age are at more risk for malnutrition (Söderström et al. 2013). The World Health Organization (WHO) has stated that geriatric populations will play a major role in global health status and challenges to health care (WHO 2008).

In India, the geriatric population is increasing (Table 2) and constitutes 7.7% of the total population (WHO 2004). Nutrition affects immunity (Lesourd 2004) and functional ability in the elderly (Stuck et al. 1999;

Galanos et al. 1994), thereby, requiring increased geriatric care. Researchers have shown that >50% of the geriatric population is underweight (Kritika et al. 2014) and >90% have below the recommended energy intake (Natarajan et al. 1993).

Table 1. A sample of the global prevalence of malnutrition

S. No.	City/Country	Risk of Malnutrition (RM)/Malnutrition (M)	References
1	Spain	RM-27%	Julio et al. 2018
2	Turkey	RM-18.6%	Nazan and Buket, 2018
3	Athens, Greece	RM-25.8%	Vassilakou et al. 2017
4	Iran	M-12.2%	Abolghasem et al. 2017
5	Japan	RM-27.1%	Kamo et al. 2019
6	Bangladesh	M-26%; RM-62%	Ferdous et al. 2009
7	China	M-12.6%	Wei et al. 2018
8	Selangor, Malaysia	RM-42.5%	Aziz et al. 2019
9	St. Petersburg, Russia	M-19%	Gurina et al. 2011
10	Ethiopia	M-21.9%	Tessfamichael et al. 2014

Table 2. A sample of Indian prevalence of malnutrition in the geriatric population

S. No.	City/State	Malnutrition (M) & Risk of Malnutrition (RM)	References
1	Vellore	M-14%; RM-49%	Vedantam et al. 2018
2	Pondicherry	M-17.9%; RM-58.7%	Krishnamoorthy et al. 2018
3	Kamrup	M-15%; RM-55%	Agarwalla et al. 2015
4	Davangere District	M-24%; RM-61%	Santosh et al. 2017
5	West Bengal	M-29.4%; RM-60.4%	Lahiri et al. 2015
6	Delhi	M-37%; RM-39%	Suri et al. 2018
7	Haryana	M-53.4%	Jamir et al. 2015
8	Lucknow	M-51%	Jingan et al. 2001
9	Allahabad	M-25%	Yadav et al. 2012
10	Kaniyambadi	M-14%	Vedantam et al. 2010

A study in rural Pondicherry showed that about 17.9% of the elderly were malnourished and about 58.7% of the elderly were at risk of malnutrition (Krishnamoorthy et al. 2018). Malnutrition status was found to be higher among individuals with no formal education, unemployed, and age >70 years. However, except for educational status ($P = 0.04$), none of the other factors were statistically significant. Studies done using the MNA questionnaire in a rural area of South India at Kaniyambadi have shown a 14% prevalence of malnutrition (Vedantam et al. 2010). In contrast, the findings of studies done in Northern India like Allahabad (25%) (Yadav et al. 2012), West Bengal (29.4%), and Haryana (53.4%) showed a higher prevalence (Lahiri et al. 2015; Jamir et al. 2015). Similar findings were reported from studies done in Vellore and West Bengal, where around 50–60% were at risk of malnutrition (Vedantam et al. 2010; Lahiri et al. 2015). The prevalence of malnutrition was higher among elderly females as compared with males in studies done at Vellore, West Bengal, and Haryana, and other developing countries like Uganda and Ethiopia. The prevalence of obesity was 32.5% in the elderly (Krishnamoorthy et al. 2018), which was similar to the findings of a study done in a rural area of Karnataka (36.7%) (Ratnaprabha et al. 2015). However, previous studies were done in rural areas of Tamil Nadu, Puducherry, and Chandigarh (Swami et al. 2005; Rajkamal et al. 2015) showed a much lesser prevalence (5-20%) of obesity (Shankar and Balamurugan 2011).

A pilot study was conducted in the geriatric urban population of Delhi, North India by our post-graduate students of diploma in health and social gerontology, using the MNA questionnaire (Mamta et al. 2018). MNA showed that 37% of the elderly were considered malnourished and 39% were taken as at risk of malnutrition. The rest 24% showed a normal nutritional status (Miu et al. 2018). Thus, malnourished status was observed to be 76% in the elderly population (Mamta et al. 2018). This higher prevalence of malnutrition emphasizes the importance of multi-disciplinary assessment, research, prevention, and treatment in the elderly.

3. Risk Factors for Malnutrition in the Elderly

The percentage of the elderly population is growing globally and may show an increase in developing countries from approximately 524 million in 2010 to about 1500 million in 2050 (Global Aging 2019). Older people are prone to malnutrition which is a multidimensional concept leading to poor health and decreased quality of life. It is a common but unrecognized disorder in the geriatric population. It is precipitated by various physiological factors (Figure 1), pathological factors, social factors, behavioral factors, and food accessibility factors (Table 3).

3.1. Physiological Factors

3.1.1. GI Tract Changes in the Elderly

During the aging loss of appetite and/or decreased food intake is frequently observed and it is termed ‘anorexia of Ageing’. After acute or chronic under-eating, the inability to appropriately increase food intake is seen in the physiological aging (Moss et al. 2012). Physiological changes in the elderly lead to decreased appetite and increased satiation. In the elderly, there is a loss of fundus compliance and rapid antral filling due to reduced secretion of nitric oxide (Morley et al. 1996). Gastroparesis may also play a role in increased postprandial satiety. Polypharmacyby the elderly especially the use of proton-pump inhibitors may also cause reduced hydrochloric acid secretion, which further delays gastric emptying. Multiple chronic illnesses in the elderly e.g., hypertension, diabetes, etc. require dietary restrictions and polypharmacy that alters food intake (Evans 2005). Dietary restrictions such as sugar, salt, and fat restriction may change food palatability. Drugs and their interactions may cause malnutrition through side effects (e.g., anorexia, nausea, and altered taste perception) as well as through altered absorption, metabolism, and excretion of nutrients. Modifications in gut microbiota, physiological of the gastrointestinal tract as well as in dietary patterns contribute to malnutrition in the elderly (Salazar et al. 2017).

3.1.2. Sensory Changes in the Elderly

Aging reduces the sensitivity to airborne chemical stimuli resulting in altered smell sensation. The inability to smell food aromas may reduce nutritional intake. Similarly, a reduced ability to detect sweet foods results in an altered taste sensation. Researchers found that the elderly have higher thresholds for perceiving sweet, bitter, salty and acid content in the diet as compared with young adults (Schiffman 1993). Taste buds show impaired cell turnover and structural abnormalities with physiological aging. Taste alteration may occur due to the reduced sense of smell, polypharmacy, illnesses and tobacco use. Taste, smell, and vision decline may reduce the enjoyment of food, dietary variety and increase anorexia. The elderly may not be able to recognize spoiled food due to taste alteration resulting in nausea, vomiting or diarrhea. These changes may also lead to depression and a vicious cycle of anorexia and weight loss (Schiffman 1993).

3.1.3. Hormonal Changes in the Elderly

Nutritional stimuli cause the release of gastrointestinal peptide hormones belonging to the appetite regulatory system. They are divided into two groups a) anorexigenic (satiety hormone) [e.g., glucagon-like peptide-1 and cholecystokinin (CCK)] or b) orexigenic (the hunger hormone) (e.g., ghrelin). Control of appetite is multifactorial, and these hormones may play an important role in the development of malnutrition in the elderly. There is a rise in satiety hormone and a fall in the hunger hormone levels in the elderly (Moss et al. 2012) thus, resulting in loss of appetite. High fasting concentrations of CCK are noted in the elderly and there is also increase sensitivity to elevated CCK (Atalayer and Astbury 2013). Similarly, oral glucose causes an enhanced glucagon-like peptide-1 response in the elderly as compared to young women, thereby explaining suppressed appetite and lower energy intake in older individuals (Ranganath et al. 1998). Anorexia of aging also shows low ghrelin levels which may reduce food intake and result in malnutrition (Atalayer and Astbury 2013). In a healthy elderly, fasting plasma leptin levels and fasting plasma insulin was found to be higher. Leptin also plays a role in the development of anorexia of aging which leads to malnutrition (Atalayer and Astbury 2013). Cytokines also play a role in malnutrition by directly acting on the gastrointestinal system or indirectly on the central nervous system. Another mechanism of action is through prostaglandins and corticotropin-releasing hormone which inhibit gastric emptying. Cytokines also interact with neuropeptides thereby inducing loss of appetite (Yeh and Schuster 1999). To summarize, hormonal mechanisms regulating energy homeostasis may change in the elderly. Changes in peripheral satiety signals including glucagon-like peptide-1, CCK, leptin, and ghrelin may influence the central control mechanisms. Coordination of energy intake control signals is modulated by these central mechanisms thus resulting in malnutrition.

3.2. Pathological Factors

Malnutrition in the elderly may be caused by pathologies that increase nutrient requirements, increase nutrient loss, reduce nutrient absorption or a combination of these factors. In clinical settings, the nutritional intake may be altered due to pure chronic starvation without inflammation (e.g., anorexia nervosa) (Mamta et al. 2018), conditions with sustained mild inflammation (e.g., cancer, rheumatoid arthritis) and acute disease with significant inflammation (Muscaritoli et al. 2010). In pathological conditions, the inflammatory response has a catabolic effect. Therefore, hypocaloric episodes in the elderly are not easy to manage due to this catabolic effect. Inflammation leads to a decrease in lean body mass and "disease-related malnutrition" (DRM). DRM is further divided into two types namely inflammatory-induced DRM within the presence of acute or chronic diseases (frailness) or as DRM without inflammation (non-cachectic).

Table 3. The factors causing malnutrition in the elderly

Pathological	Food accessibility	Behavioral factors	Social factors
• Multiple Medications	• Lack of mobility	• Depression	• Social isolation
• Multiple Morbidities (Diabetes, Hypertension, Stroke)	• Physical disability	• Anxiety	• Poor social integration
• Surgical Procedures	• Lack of knowledge (Food, cooking, nutrition)	• Poor cognitive function	• Education
• Helicobacter pylori infection	• Inability to shop or prepare meals	• Chronic alcoholism	• Marital status
• Diarrheal diseases	• Smaller/less frequent meals	• Smoking	• Financial Status
• Malabsorption Syndrome	• Low fiber diet/ constipation	• Lack of exercise	• Living arrangements
• Hospitalization	• Low fluid intake/dehydratio n	• Bereavement	• Gender
• Neurodegenerative disorders	• Needs feeding/supervisi on	• Dementia	• Leisure Activities
• Malignancy	• Failure to reach food, cutlery, or packages	• Stress	• Pension
• Anorexia Nervosa	• Food availability	• Chronic pain	• Number of cohabitants
• Chronic & end-stage disease	• Food expenditure	• Sleep disorders	• Perceived satisfaction with social support

The pathophysiology of common neurological and neurodegenerative disorders in the elderly is inflammation (Cederholm et al. 2017). Therefore, these disorders may lead to malnutrition. Significant pathological risk factors for malnutrition in elderly besides inflammation is polypharmacy (Prell and Perner 2018), multiple morbidities, surgery, malabsorption syndromes, helicobacter infection, diarrheal diseases, general Parkinson's disease, cognitive decline, dementia, institutionalization, impaired motor skills, sensory, and cognitive decline, etc.(Dumic et al. 2019).

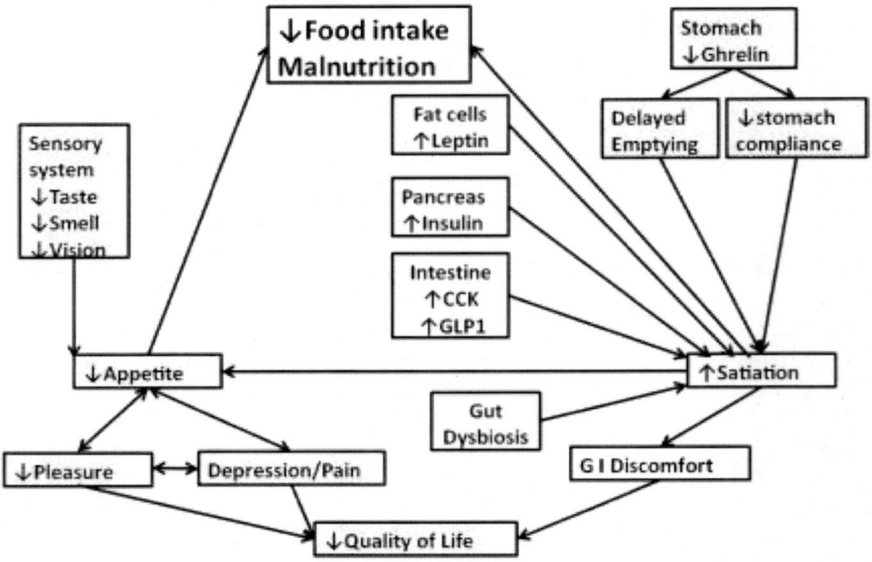

Figure 1. Physiological factors causing malnutrition in the elderly.

3.2.1. Food Accessibility Factors

Food accessibility factors causing malnutrition in the elderly are limited accessibility of a balanced and culturally relevant diet. Other factors that play a role are limited ability to acquire food, food hygiene, and socially acceptable ways of accessing food (Wolfe et al. 2003). The elderly with dependency have diet issues that may lead to malnutrition. Diet compromises due to financial reasons include a reduced number of meals, replacement of certain types of foods for others and choosing between food and medicine. In the geriatric population, diet quality compromise is common, sometimes quality is preserved but quantity is compromised. Various food accessibility factors causing malnutrition in the elderly are listed in Table 3. Nutrition and dietetics services in the elderly should recognize food accessibility factors and provide services to cover those needs (Wolfe et al. 2003).

3.3. Behavioral Factors

Depression and malnutrition are prevalent among the geriatric population and seem to be strongly associated. There is a vicious circle between depression and deficiency disease. Depression leads to appetite and weight changes that result in malnutrition, and poor nutrition predisposes old individuals to depression. A study conducted in our department also shows that pain, depression, and anxiety are associated with malnutrition in the geriatric population (Mamta et al. 2018). Changes in the diet are associated with anxiety or stress e.g., bereavement has been shown to be associated with negative effects on eating behaviors and nutrient intake. Similarly, smokers also show a negative association with the risk of malnutrition. Smoking status in chronic obstructive pulmonary disease outpatients is a significant independent risk factor for malnutrition (Collins et al. 2011). Anorexia of aging is another component of geriatric syndromes which is associated with a higher risk of malnutrition. Anorexia may increase the risk of qualitative malnutrition, due to reduced intake of single nutrients, like proteins and vitamins in the early stages but in late stages, it leads to quantitative malnutrition as well (Muscaritoli et al. 2010). Selective deficiency malnutrition is additionally associated with sarcopenia and other negative health outcomes with increased morbidity and mortality (Rahman et al. 2008; Francesco et al. 2010; Martone et al. 2013). The cornerstone of treating anorexia is still nutrition rehabilitation which should be initiated immediately (Arlington 2006).

3.4. Socioeconomic Factors

Various social scientists have shown that there is an association between socioeconomic status and diet (Megabiaw and Rahman 2013; Rahman 2016; Rahman et al. 2016). Socioeconomic factors that contribute to poorer diets in the elderly are poor social integration, lack of education, marital status, bereavement, pension, living arrangements and frequency of networking with friends. Researchers have reported a positive role of resilience and self-efficacy on diet quality among the elderly. The pattern of associations between socioeconomic factors and diet quality shows the gendered difference in the elderly. But having greater emotional support positively relates to both men's and women's diet quality (Bloom et al. 2017). Higher overall participation in leisure activities, including both social and cognitive activities, was positively related to better quality diets. Individuals with no family income had double the risk of malnutrition as compared to those who earned at least three minimum wages. The risk for malnutrition was inversely related to an increased number of people living with the elderly (Damião et al. 2017). To conclude, a multidisciplinary approach is needed to manage modifiable risk factors and prevent complications of malnutrition in the geriatric population

4. Outcomes of Malnutrition in the Elderly

Age-related malnutrition is associated with various physiological, pathological, behavioral, psychological, socioeconomic and food accessibility risk factors (Table 3). There is a vicious cycle of malnutrition and geriatric syndromes in the elderly. Therefore, early detection of malnutrition should be given due importance in the geriatric assessment to prevent and treat unhealthy outcomes of malnutrition in the geriatric population. Outcomes of malnutrition in the elderly include poor physical health, poor bone health, poor mental health, decreased quality of life and increase mortality (Figure 2).

4.1. Malnutrition and Physical Health

Outcomes of malnutrition include poor general physical health, poor immune function, delayed recovery, increased morbidity, and mortality, etc. (Ahmed and Haboubi 2010; 2017; Rahman et al. 2019). Despite under treatment of health professionals, 25% of at-risk malnourished elderly patients do not receive nutritional counseling (Orrevall et al. 2009), which should play a major role in geriatric treatment programs.

4.2. Immune System and Malnutrition

Malnutrition profoundly affects immune responses in the geriatric population. There are three stages of immune Ageing. Stage 1: Healthy aging- It is primary immune aging in the healthy elderly with no nutritional deficiency and changes in T cells population. The T-cell function is reduced only in the elderly >90 years of age. Stage 2: Common aging- It is a secondary immune aging common in the elderly with micronutrient deficiency and correctable by nutritional supplementation. These immune responses may also be enhanced by the supplementation of the elderly who have no micronutrient deficiency. Stage 3: Pathological aging- It is tertiary immune aging in patients with protein-energy deficiency. In these patients, a decrease in immune response may result in the depletion of nutritional reserves during illness and increased frailty. Therefore, malnutrition has immune aging responses in the elderly requiring nutritional therapy. Elderly, who do not have nutrient deficits may also benefit from nutrition supplementation resulting in the promotion of healthy aging and extension of the lifespan (Lesourd 2006).

4.3. Wound Healing and Malnutrition

Wound healing processes form a cascade of inflammation, proliferation, and remodeling. Both micronutrients and macronutrients are essential in all three phases of wound healing. Researchers have shown that for DNA synthesis, cell division, and proliferation minerals like zinc and iron play an important role. For structural processes such as collagen synthesis and strength as well as re-epithelialization, proteins, iron, zinc, vitamin-A, and vitamin-C are important (Barchitta et al. 2019). Immune processes e.g., antibody response, leukocyte migration to the wound site, disposal of waste products produced by leukocytes, size as well as a number of lymphocytes and killer T-cells, are altered by the status of these nutrients in elderly (Harris and Fraser 2004). Therefore, malnutrition leads to poor wound healing and delay in post-surgical recovery.

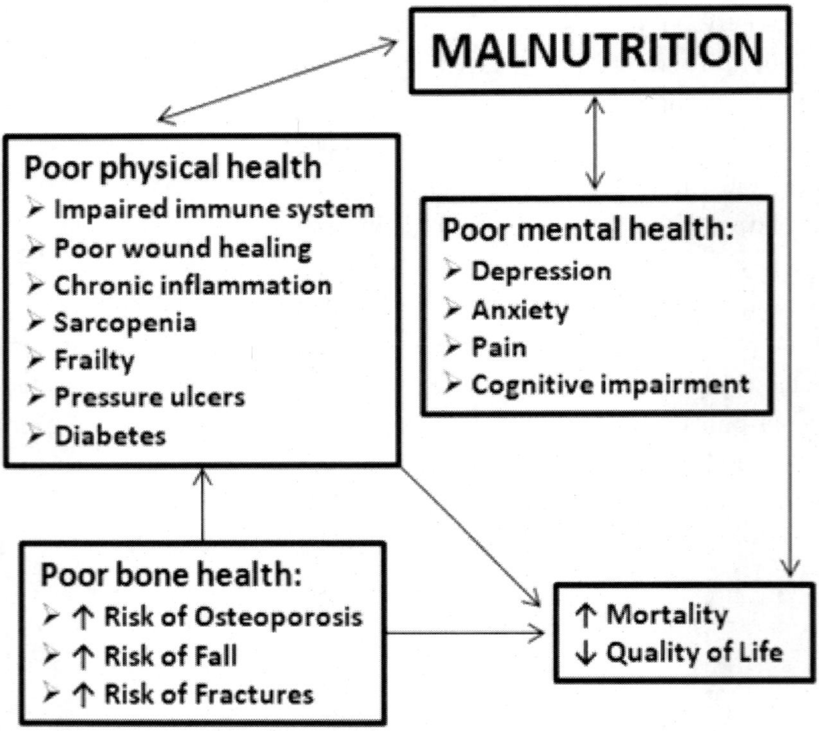

Figure 2. Outcomes of malnutrition in the elderly.

Carbohydrates provide glucose for fibroblastic production and movement, leukocyte activity, mitosis, protein synthesis, hormones secretion, and growth factors secretion during wound healing (Barchitta et al. 2019). Glucose provides calories needed for the inflammatory process and cellular activity, angiogenesis and collagen deposition. Therefore, calories may need to be increased by 50% for wound recovery (Molnar et al. 2014). Fats are calories providers, constituents of cell membranes, prostaglandins precursors and contributors to cell signaling pathways (Harris and Fraser 2004). Therefore, their deficiency state leads to impaired immunity and wound healing. Protein-energy malnutrition (PEM) may also impair immunity with resultant recurrent infections (Rahman 2019; Rahman and Rahman 2019; Rahman et al. 2019). Proteins are important constituents of immune cells and their deficiency leads to impaired inflammatory response and delayed progression to the proliferative phase of wound healing. PEM delays angiogenesis in the proliferative stage and reduces fibroblastic activity collagen synthesis and maturation in the remodeling stage thus resulting in the non-healing wound (Harris and Fraser 2004). PEM also stimulate cytokines production, induction of inflammation, immunodeficiency, and anemia. Chronic wound exudation and edema lead to further loss of proteins and complications. Therefore, dietary proteins may need to be increased by 2.5 times for wound recovery (Molnar et al. 2014).

Vitamins are also essential for wound healing. Vitamin-C plays an important role in immune response, cell mitosis, monocyte migration, and transformation into macrophages during the inflammatory phase of wound healing. It removes free radicals, increases collagen production and wound strength. Vitamin-C deficiencies also cause increased capillary fragility and non-healing wounds (Harris and Fraser 2004). Similarly, vitamin-A improves cell-mediated immunity and collagen synthesis. It reduces susceptibility to infections and increases collagen and granulation tissue development in the proliferative stages of wound healing. Vitamin-B assists in leukocyte formation and collagen matrix synthesis. It is an essential cofactor in enzyme activity. It improves antibody formation and blood cell function. Thus, vitamin-B deficiency decreases immunity. Nutritional anemia is seen in the elderly with vitamin-B12, folic acid, and vitamin-C deficiency. Vitamin-K deficiency contributes to decreased coagulation. Therefore, vitamin deficiencies impair the wound healing process (Harris and Fraser 2004). Similarly, minerals like iron transport oxygen to the tissues which are necessary for collagen synthesis. Therefore, iron and copper deficiency are the causes of nutritional anemia and delayed wound healing in the elderly. Zinc produces antibodies and activates lymphocytes in the inflammatory phase of wound healing. Zinc stimulates the enzyme activities and is necessary for the stability of membrane and the maturation of collagen in wound healing. Therefore, zinc deficiency may reduce immune response, wound strength and increase the risk of repeated infections (Lin et al. 2017).

4.4. Inflammation and Malnutrition

Nutrients play an important role in both promoting and preventing inflammatory processes. Inflammation leads to increased nitrogen excretion, increased resting energy expenditure, impaired protein utilization, anorexia and impaired utilization of nutrients thereby leading to malnutrition. There is a vicious cycle between malnutrition and inflammation. Management of inflammation is better if nutritional requirements continue to be met throughout the treatment process (Carriere et al. 2008).

4.5. Sarcopenia and Malnutrition

The European working group on sarcopenia in older people defines sarcopenia as loss of muscle mass, loss of strength, functionality, or both in the elderly (Cruz-Jentoft et al. 2010). Sarcopenia is divided into primary and secondary sarcopenia. Primary sarcopenia is an idiopathic, progressive, and related to intrinsic aging factors. Secondary sarcopenia is related to multiple extrinsic factors. Similarly, International Guideline Consensus Committee divided malnutrition into three subtypes (a) starvation-related malnutrition without inflammation, (b) chronic disease-related malnutrition with inflammation e.g., sarcopenia and (c) acute disease or injury-related malnutrition with inflammation (Jensen et al. 2010). Although malnutrition and sarcopenia have different pathophysiology but common symptoms e.g., abnormal bodyweight or inactivity (Jeejeebhoy 2012; Vandewoude et al. 2012). This research coined a new term, “malnutrition-sarcopenia syndrome”, consisting of both malnutrition and sarcopenia (Wei et al. 2017). Thus, there is a vicious cycle between sarcopenia and malnutrition and both are a process as well as an outcome.

4.6. Frailty and Malnutrition

Frailty could be a geriatric syndrome with an associate elevated risk of declines in health and performance among older adults. Fried et al. suggested labeling of frailty on the basis of three out of five criteria of compromised energetic: low grip strength, low energy, slowed walking speed, low physical activity, and/or unintentional weight loss (Fried et al. 2001). A pre-frail stage elderly are at higher risk of progressing to frailty and are diagnosed if one or two criteria are present. Frailty and malnutrition are related but distinct conditions in the elderly. The risk for malnutrition and malnutrition are correlated with pre-frailty and frailty (Tseng et al. 1995). Adverse health outcomes attributed to malnutrition often appear more likely to be associated with frailty. There is an inverse association between micronutrients and/or macronutrients and frailty. Diet quality is also inversely associated with the risk of being frail. Thus, malnutrition outcomes include frailty and there is evidence that frailty outcomes include malnutrition.

4.7. Pressure Ulcers and Malnutrition

A localized injury to the skin and underlying tissue over a bony prominence is called pressure ulcers. There is impaired perfusion, progressive destruction, and necrosis of the underlying tissues (Emily 2014). It is common in the elderly with physical or cognitive impairments, multiple comorbidities, prolonged hospitalization, spinal cord injury, etc. In pressure ulcer healing, tissue viability and repair depend on nutrition and hydration (Posthauer et al. 2015). Therefore, malnutrition predisposes to pressure ulcer formation.

4.8. Diabetes and Malnutrition

Researchers have reported that minorities living in urban areas of the US are prone to malnutrition and have increased rates of diabetes (Jen et al. 2007). Malnutrition-related diabetes mellitus is a rare type of diabetes associated with long-term malnutrition. This type of diabetes is characterized by insulinopenia, insulin resistance, hyperglycemia, and failure of the β-cells in the pancreas. Diabetic elderly may also have comorbidities like dyslipidemia, and a cardiovascular disease that may impact their nutritional requirements resulting in malnutrition. Malnutrition is generally associated with undernutrition but it can also result from over nutrition, obesity, and diabetes. Elderly type 2 diabetics with malnutrition have higher mortality risk due to any cause vs. those without nutrition deficiencies. Diabetes-related malnutrition complicates treatment plans and negatively impacts patient outcomes, such as recovery, complications, re-hospitalizations, and rehabilitation.

4.9. Malnutrition and Mental Health

Various researchers have shown an association between psychological and nutritional problems in the elderly. A high prevalence of malnutrition, depression, anxiety, pain, and cognitive decline are reported among the elderly.

4.9.1. Depression and Malnutrition

Malnutrition can induce depression because of psychological vulnerability in the elderly (Wada 2000). Although researchers have shown a correlation between malnutrition and depression (Tamura et al. 2013; Lizaka et al. 2008; Smoliner et al. 2009; Ferdous et al. 2009; Kulnik and

Elmadfa 2008; Saka et al. 2010; Feldblum et al. 2007; Rodríguez-Tadeo et al. 2012; Vanderwee et al. 2010; Yoshimura et al. 2013), however, the causal relationship between depression and nutritional status is still unclear (Singh et al. 2014). One of the serious unfavorable effects and correctable causes of malnutrition is depression (Vellas et al. 2001; Saletti et al. 2000; Suominen et al. 2005). Malnourished patients have higher depression scores (Morley and Kraenzle 1994; Blaum et al. 1995). A pilot study by our gerontology students reported that malnutrition and depressive symptoms have a high prevalence among the urban geriatric population in Delhi, India (Mamta et al. 2018). Malnutrition produces various physiological impairments such as reduced mobility, muscle pain, and weakness, etc. which may increase the prevalence of depressive symptoms. Nutritional deficiency leading to cachexia, dehydration, electrolytes impairment and multivitamin deficiency, is frequently associated with depression (Heseker et al. 1995). In the elderly, folic acid deficiency may result in psychiatric symptoms. The biogenic theory of affective disorders explains the relationship between folate deficiency, pyridoxine deficiency, and mood disorder. Therefore, malnutrition and depression are unfavorable outcomes for one another in the elderly.

4.9.2. Anxiety and Malnutrition

A pilot study in our department reported anxiety levels (54%) to have a positive association with malnutrition (76%) among the elderly population in Delhi (Mamta et al. 2018). Anxiety and malnutrition are comorbid entities e.g., magnesium deficiency may lead to irritability whereas selenium deficiency alters the mood. Similarly, omega-3 polyunsaturated fatty acids deficiency also increases the risk of anxiety. The relationship between anxiety and malnutrition is complex and reciprocal. Anxiety may be associated with alteration in food intake e.g., binge eating, seeking “comfort foods”, decreased food intake or fasting. Nature of stressor, the intensity of anxiety, duration of anxiety, gender and cultural differences in eating habits may play a role in the development of malnutrition. The effects of acute and chronic anxiety may also be different from the nutritional status of the elderly (Bellisle et al. 1990).

4.9.3. Pain and Malnutrition

Various studies have shown that nutritional status can be associated with pain perception. Takahashi et al. (Takahashi et al. 2014) reported that malnourished cancer patients have significantly higher pain intensities as compared to patients in the normal-nutrition group. Pain intensities and Nutrition Risk Screening 2002 (NRS 2002) scores show a significant association. These results suggest that an increase in the NRS 2002 score is associated with an increase in pain intensity in cancer patients. Malnutrition may also lead to poor pain management in cancer patients. We also reported that malnourished elders have a higher risk to develop moderate to severe pain. Similarly, other researchers have reported that the prevalence of malnutrition and the intensity of somatic symptoms as well as psychological stress are high among lung cancer patients. The lung cancer patients at risk of malnutrition show significant pain as compare to patients with a normal nutritional status (Mamta et al. 2018). Therefore, maintaining a healthy nutritional status is important to manage painful conditions in the elderly (Chabowski et al. 2018).

4.9.4. Cognitive Impairment and Malnutrition

Malnutrition plays a role in the progression of psychological imbalance in the elderly. There is a vicious cycle between cognitive impairment and nutritional status (Lee et al. 2009; Rahman et al. 2009). Various factors which affect malnutrition also alter cognitive state, such as oral health-related problems (Wojszel 2006). Generally, malnutrition results in functional impairment in activities of daily living that require higher care. Patients affected by serious cognitive impairment show poor nutritional state, poor functional conditions and increased morbidity/mortality (Malara et al. 2014).

4.9.5. Malnutrition and Bone Health

Malnutrition impacts bone health and increases the risk of osteoporosis, falls and fractures. Many nutrients in addition to vitamin-D and calcium, may impact skeletal mass and bone mineral density (Siddique et al. 2017). Therefore, dietary interventions or supplementations of these nutrients or targeting eating behaviors have shown positive results.

4.9.5.1. Osteoporosis

Malnutrition, particularly protein undernutrition, may lower bone mass and alter muscle strength resulting in an osteoporotic fracture. It may also increase the medical complications after an osteoporotic fracture. Rizzoli and Bonjour (Rizzoli and Bonjour 1999) reported that osteoporotic hip fractures in the involvement of the elderly show of an insulin-like growth factor 1 (IGF-I) system. Protein supplementation in the presence of adequate calcium and vitamin-D raises IGF-I levels. Thus, improving hip fracture recovery and proximal femur bone mineral density within the year following the fracture. Therefore, two nutrients of calcium and vitamin-D are essential for bone health. Loss of bone mass and induction of osteoporosis is related to low supplies of calcium. Calcium supplementation reduces the rate of bone loss in osteoporotic patients. Vitamin-D insufficiency is also common in the geriatric population. The major causes of vitamin-D deficiency in the elderly are malnutrition, decreased renal hydroxylation of vitamin-D, reduced exposure to sunlight and a decline in the synthesis of vitamin-D in the skin (Gennari 2001; Siddique et al. 2017).

4.9.5.2. Falls

Various researchers have shown that malnutrition is associated with falls or able to predict falls of older people (Johnson 2003; Vivanti, Ward, and Haines 2011; Meijers et al. 2012; Neyens et al. 2013). The level of nutritional risk is an important determinant of falls along with leg strength and balance among frail older adults (Rodríguez-Tadeo et al. 2012). Malnutrition and impaired mobility are modifiable factors related to falls. Therefore, the management of malnutrition and impaired mobility are important preventive strategies for a potential fall in the elderly (Meijers et al. 2012).

4.9.5.3. Fractures

In geriatric patients with hip fractures, malnutrition is common. Malnutrition may contribute to the fractures in the elderly through two mechanisms: (a) sarcopenia which increases the risk of falls thereby increasing the risk of fracture (b) osteoporosis which reduces the resistance of bones to trauma and increasing the risk of fracture (Huang et al. 1996). Treatment of modifiable factor-like malnutrition improves the outcomes of hip fracture surgery, such as pressure ulcers (Hommel et al. 2007). An increase in dietary vitamin-D and calcium intake in the elderly can decrease fracture risk especially in regions where fracture incidence in high (Prentice 2004).

4.9.6. Malnutrition and Quality of Life

Malnutrition is underestimated in the geriatric population. It affects the quality of life morbidity and mortality rate among the elderly. Nutritional interventions can lead to significant improvements in both physical and mental aspects of quality of life (Rasheed and Woods 2013). Researchers have shown that malnutrition increases the duration and/or cost of hospitalization as well as rehabilitation. It increases morbidity and mortality rates in the geriatric population. Reported adverse health outcomes attributed to poor nutrition usually seem additional probably to be related to physical frailty (Wei et al. 2018), however, frailty could also be the associated outcome of malnutrition.

CONCLUSION

Malnutrition often remains underestimated, undetected or untreated in the elderly. While some risk factors of malnutrition in the elderly are non-modifiable but many others are modifiable and treatable. Malnutrition in the elderly can be the result of physiological, psychological, and socioeconomic factors. Frail elderly with nutritional counseling and supplementation may become less prone to malnutrition and its complications. Therefore, elderly health care and health policies must take nutritional status into account especially during acute and/or chronic health challenges. Modifiable determinants of nutritional status should be targeted in the home, hospital, and long-term care settings are need of the hour for the elderly. Malnutrition may also be used as a prognostic factor for accessing the outcome of morbidity in the elderly. Identifying and treating nutrition issues early in the elderly can promote good health and increased longevity.

REFERENCES

AbolghasemGorji, H., Alikhani, M., Mohseni, M., Moradi-Joo, M., Ziaiifar, H. & Moosavi, A. (2017). The Prevalence of Malnutrition in Iranian Elderly: A Review Article. *Iranian Journal of Public Health*, 46 (12), 1603-10.

Ahmed, T. & Haboubi, N. (2010). Assessment and Management of Nutrition in Older People and Its Importance to Health. *Clinical Interventions in Aging*, 5, 207–16.

Al-Rasheed, R., Alrasheedi, R., Al Johani, R., Alrashidi, H., Almaimany, B., Alshalawi, B., Kelantan, A., Banjar, G., Alzaher, A. & Alqadheb, A. (2018). Malnutrition in Elderly and Its Relation to Depression. *International Journal of Community Medicine and Public Health*, 5 (6), 2156–60. https://doi.org/10.18203/2394-6040.ijcmph20181974.

Arlington, V. A. (2006). Treatment of Patients with Eating Disorders, Third Edition. In *APA Practice Guidelines for the Treatment of Psychiatric Disorders: Comprehensive Guidelines and Guideline Watches*, by American Psychiatric Association, 1st ed. Vol. 1, American Psychiatric Association. https://doi.org/10.1176/appi.books.9780890423363.138660.

Atalayer, D. & Astbury, N. M. (2013). Anorexia of Aging and Gut Hormones. *Aging and Disease*, 4 (5), 264–75. https://doi.org/10.14336/AD.2013.0400264.

Aziz, N. S. A., Teng, N. M. F. & Zaman, M. K. (2019). Geriatric Nutrition Risk Index is Comparable to the Mini Nutritional Assessment for Assessing Nutritional Status in Elderly Hospitalized Patients. *Clinical Nutrition ESPEN*, 29, 77–85. doi: 10.1016/j.clnesp.2018.12.002.

Barchitta, M., Maugeri, A., Favara, G., Magnano San Lio, R., Evola, G., Agodi, A. & Basile, G. (2019). Nutrition and Wound Healing: An Overview Focusing on the Beneficial Effects of Curcumin. *International Journal of Molecular Sciences*, 20 (5). https://doi.org/10.3390/ijms20051119.

Bellisle, F., Louis-Sylvestre, J., Linet, N., Rocaboy, B., Dalle, B., Cheneau, F., L'Hinoret, D. & Guyot, L. (1990). Anxiety and Food Intake in Men. *Psychosomatic Medicine*, 52 (4), 452–57.

Blaum, C. S., Fries, B. E. & Fiatarone, M. A. (1995). Factors Associated with Low Body Mass Index and Weight Loss in Nursing Home Residents. *The Journals of Gerontology. Series A, Biological Sciences and Medical Sciences*, 50 (3), M162-168. https://doi.org/10.1093/gerona/50a.3.m162.

Bloom, I., Edwards, M., Jameson, K. A., Syddall, H. E., Dennison, E., Gale, C. R., Baird, J., Cooper, C., Aihie Sayer, A. & Robinson, S. (2017). Influences on Diet Quality in Older Age: The Importance of Social Factors. *Age and Ageing*, 46 (2), 277–83. https://doi.org/10.1093/ageing/afw180.

Carriere, I., Dupuy, A. M., Lacroux, A., Cristol, J. P., Delcourt, C. & Pathologies Oculaires Liées à l'Age Study Group. (2008). Biomarkers of Inflammation and Malnutrition Associated with Early Death in Healthy Elderly People. *Journal of the American Geriatrics Society*, 56 (5), 840–46. https://doi.org/10.1111/j.1532-5415.2008.01677.x.

Cederholm, T., Barazzoni, R., Austin, P., Ballmer, P., Biolo, G., Bischoff, S. C., Compher, S., et al. 2017. ESPEN Guidelines on Definitions and Terminology of Clinical Nutrition. *Clinical Nutrition (Edinburgh, Scotland)*, 36 (1), 49–64. https://doi.org/10.1016/j.clnu.2016.09.004.

Cereda, E. (2012). Mini Nutritional Assessment. *Current Opinion in Clinical Nutrition and Metabolic Care*, 15 (1), 29–41. https://doi.org/10.1097/MCO.0b013e32834d7647.

Chabowski, M., Polański, J., Jankowska-Polańska, B., Janczak, D. & Rosińczuk, J. (2018). Is Nutritional Status Associated with the Level of Anxiety, Depression, and Pain in Patients with Lung Cancer? *Journal of Thoracic Disease*, 10 (4), 2303–10. https://doi.org/10.21037/jtd.2018.03.108.

Collins, P. F., Stratton, R. J. & Elia, M. (2011).The Influence of Smoking Status on Malnutrition Risk and 1-year Mortality in Outpatients with Chronic Obstructive Pulmonary Disease. *Journal of Human Nutrition and Dietetics*, 24 (4), 382-383. https://doi.org/10.1111/j.1365-277X.2011.01177_11.x.

Cruz-Jentoft A, J., Baeyens, J, P., Bauer, J. M., Boirie, Y., Cederholm, T., Landi, F., Martin, F. C., et al. (2010). Sarcopenia: European Consensus on Definition and Diagnosis: Report of the European Working Group on Sarcopenia in Older People. *Age and Ageing*, 39 (4), 412–23. https://doi.org/10.1093/ageing/afq034.

Damião, R., da Silva Santos, A., Matijasevich, A. & Menezes, P. R. (2017). Factors Associated with Risk of Malnutrition in the Elderly in South-Eastern Brazil. *Revista Brasileira De Epidemiologia = Brazilian Journal of Epidemiology*, 20 (4), 598–610. https://doi.org/10.1590/1980-5497201700040004.

Tessfamichael, D., Gete, A. A. & Wassie, M. M. (2014). High Prevalence of Undernutrition among Elderly People in Northwest Ethiopia: A Cross-Sectional Study. *Journal of Nutritional Health and Food Science*, 2 (3), 1-5. http://dx.doi.org/10.15226/jnhfs.2014.00131.

Dumic, I., Nordin, T., Jecmenica, M., Lalosevic, M. S., Milosavljevic, T. & Milovanovic, T. (2019). Gastrointestinal Tract Disorders in Older Age. *Canadian Journal of Gastroenterology & Hepatology*, 6757524. https://doi.org/10.1155/2019/6757524.

Elia, M. (2000). British Association for Parenteral and Enteral Nutrition, and Advisory Group on Malnutrition. *Guidelines for Detection and Management of Malnutrition*. Maidenhead: BAPEN.

Evans, C. (2005). Malnutrition in the Elderly: A Multifactorial Failure to Thrive. *The Permanente Journal*, 9 (3), 38–41.

Feldblum, I., German, L., Castel, H., Harman-Boehm, I., Bilenko, N., Eisinger, M., Fraser, D. & Shahar, D. R. (2007). Characteristics of Undernourished Older Medical Patients and the Identification of Predictors for Undernutrition Status. *Nutrition Journal*, 6, 37. https://doi.org/10.1186/1475-2891-6-37.

Ferdous, T., Kabir, Z. N., Wahlin, A., Streatfield, K. & Cederholm, T. (2009). The Multidimensional Background of Malnutrition among Rural Older Individuals in Bangladesh-a Challenge for the Millennium Development Goal. *Public Health Nutrition*, 12 (12), 2270–78. https://doi.org/10.1017/S1368980009005096.

Fried, L. P., Tangen, C. M., Walston, J., Newman, A. B., Hirsch, C., Gottdiener, J., Seeman, T., et al. (2001). Frailty in Older Adults: Evidence for a Phenotype. *The Journals of Gerontology. Series A, Biological Sciences and Medical Sciences*, 56 (3), M146-156. https://doi.org/10.1093/gerona/56.3.m146.

Galanos, A. N., Pieper, C. F., Cornoni-Huntley, J. C., Bales, C. W. & Fillenbaum, G. G. (1994). Nutrition and Function: Is There a Relationship between Body Mass Index and the Functional Capabilities of Community-Dwelling Elderly? *Journal of the American Geriatrics Society*, 42 (4), 368–73.

Gennari, C. (2001). Calcium and Vitamin D Nutrition and Bone Disease of the Elderly. *Public Health Nutrition*, 4 (2B), 547–59.

Gil-Montoya, J. A., Ponce, G., Sánchez Lara, I., Barrios, R., Llodra, J. C. & Bravo, M. (2013). Association of the Oral Health Impact Profile with Malnutrition Risk in Spanish Elders. *Archives of Gerontology and Geriatrics*, 57 (3), 398–402. https://doi.org/10.1016/j.archger. 2013.05.002.

Global Aging. (2019). Accessed June 6, 2019. https://www.nia.nih.gov/research/dbsr/global-aging.

Gurina, N. A., Frolova, E. V. & Degryse, J. M. (2011). A roadmap of aging in Russia: the prevalence of frailty in community-dwelling older adults in the St. Petersburg district-the "Crystal" study. *Journal of the American Geriatrics Society*, 59 (6), 980-88. doi: 10.1111/j.1532-5415.2011.03448.x. Epub 2011 Jun 7.

Hakim, M. A. & Rahman, A. (2016). Health and nutritional condition of street children of Dhaka city: an empirical study in Bangladesh. *Science Journal of Public Health*, 4 (1), 6-9.

Hasan, N., Ashraf, M. & Rahman, A. (2016). Effects of information communication technology (ICT) in the childhood developments and lives of disabilities: A multivariate analysis. *Science Journal of Public Health*, 4 (1), 28-37. https://doi.org/10.11648/j.sjph.s.2016040101.15.

Harris, C. L. & Fraser, C. (2004). Malnutrition in the Institutionalized Elderly: The Effects on Wound Healing. *Ostomy/Wound Management*, 50 (10), 54–63.

Heseker, H., Kübler, W., Pudel, V. & Westenhöfer, J. (1995). Interaction of Vitamins with Mental Performance. *Bibliotheca Nutritio Et Dieta.*, 52, 43–55.

Hickson, M. (2006). Malnutrition and Ageing. *Postgraduate Medical Journal*, 82 (963), 2–8. https://doi.org/10.1136/pgmj.2005.037564.

Hommel, A., Bjorkelund, K. B., Thorngren, K. G. & Ulander, K. (2007). Nutritional Status among Patients with Hip Fracture in Relation to Pressure Ulcers. *Clinical Nutrition (Edinburgh, Scotland)*, 26 (5), 589–96. https://doi.org/10.1016/j.clnu.2007.06.003.

Huang, Z., Himes, J. H. & McGovern, P. G. (1996). Nutrition and Subsequent Hip Fracture Risk among a National Cohort of White Women. *American Journal of Epidemiology*, 144 (2), 124–34. https://doi.org/10.1093/oxfordjournals.aje.a008899.

Yadav, N., Ravindra, R., Sharma, S., Singh, A., Mishra, M., Dubey, J., et al. (2012). Dietary Habits and Nutritional Status of Elderly Living in Urban Areas of Allahabad District. *Indian Journal of Preventive & Social Medicine*, 43 (1), 81-6.

Lizaka, S., Tadaka, E. & Sanada, H. (2008). Comprehensive Assessment of Nutritional Status and Associated Factors in the Healthy, Community-Dwelling Elderly. *Geriatrics & Gerontology International*, 8 (1), 24–31. https://doi.org/10.1111/j.1447-0594.2008.00443.x.

Jamir, L., Kalaivani, M., Nongkynrih, B., Misra, P. & Gupta, S. K. (2015). Anthropometric Characteristics and Undernutrition among Older Persons in a Rural Area of Northern India. *Asia-Pacific Journal of*

Public Health, 27 (2), NP2246-2258. https://doi.org/10.1177/1010539513490191.

Jeejeebhoy, K. N. (2012). Malnutrition, Fatigue, Frailty, Vulnerability, Sarcopenia and Cachexia: Overlap of Clinical Features. *Current Opinion in Clinical Nutrition and Metabolic Care*, 15 (3), 213–19. https://doi.org/10.1097/MCO.0b013e328352694f.

Jen, K. L., Brogan, K., Washington, O. G., Flack, J. M. & Artinian, N. T. (2007). Poor Nutrient Intake and High Obese Rate in an Urban African American Population with Hypertension. *Journal of the American College of Nutrition*, 26 (1), 57–65.

Jensen, G. L., Mirtallo, J., Compher, C., Dhaliwal, R., Forbes, A., Grijalba, R. F., Hardy, G., et al. (2010). Adult Starvation and Disease-Related Malnutrition: A Proposal for Etiology-Based Diagnosis in the Clinical Practice Setting from the International Consensus Guideline Committee. *JPEN. Journal of Parenteral and Enteral Nutrition*, 34 (2), 156–59. https://doi.org/10.1177/0148607110361910.

Johnson, C. S. (2003). The Association between Nutritional Risk and Falls among Frail Elderly. *The Journal of Nutrition, Health & Aging*, *7* (4), 247–50.

Julio, M. P. M., Clavero, A. E. & Soler, M. L. M. (2018). Nutritional status and factors associated with non-institutionalized people over 75 years of age. *Revista Brasileira De Enfermagem*, 71 (3), 1007–12. https://doi.org/10.1590/0034-7167-2017-0207.

Kaiser, M. J., Bauer, J. M., Rämsch, C., Uter, W., Guigoz, Y., Cederholm, T., Thomas, D. R., et al. (2010). Frequency of Malnutrition in Older Adults: A Multinational Perspective Using the Mini Nutritional Assessment. *Journal of the American Geriatrics Society*, 58 (9), 1734–38. https://doi.org/10.1111/j.1532-5415.2010.03016.x.

Kamo, T, Ishii, H., Suzuki, K. & Nishida, Y. (2019). The Impact of Malnutrition on Efficacy of Resistance Training in Community-Dwelling Older Adults. *Physiotherapy Research International*, 24 (1), e1755. doi: 10.1002/pri.1755.

Kansal, D., Baliga, S. S., Kruthika, K. & Mallapur, M. D. (2016). Nutritional Assessment among Elderly Population of Rural Belagavi:

A Cross-Sectional Study. *International Journal of Medical Science and Public Health*, 5 (7), 1496–99.

Krishnamoorthy, Y., Vijayageetha, M., Kumar, S. G., Rajaa, S. & Rehman, T. (2018). Prevalence of Malnutrition and Its Associated Factors among Elderly Population in Rural Puducherry Using Mini-Nutritional Assessment Questionnaire. *Journal of Family Medicine and Primary Care*, 7 (6), 1429. https://doi.org/10.4103/jfmpc.jfmpc_22_18.

Kritika, D., Semwal, J., Vyas, S., Juyal, R. & Sati, H. C. (2014). Nutritional Status and Associated Comorbidities among the Elderly in Doiwala Block, Dehradun. *Indian Journal of Community Health*, 26 (Supp 2), 197–203.

Kulnik, D. & Elmadfa, I. (2008). Assessment of the Nutritional Situation of Elderly Nursing Home Residents in Vienna. *Annals of Nutrition & Metabolism*, 52, Suppl 1, 51–53. https://doi.org/10.1159/000115350.

Lahiri, S., Biswas, A., Santra, S. & Lahiri, S. K. (2015). Assessment of Nutritional Status among Elderly Population in a Rural Area of West Bengal, India. *International Journal of Medical Science and Public Health*, 4 (4), 569–72.

Francesco, L., Laviano, A. & Cruz-Jentoft, A. J. (2010). The Anorexia of Aging: Is It a Geriatric Syndrome? *Journal of the American Medical Directors Association*, 11 (3), 153–56. https://doi.org/10.1016/j.jamda.2009.09.003.

Lee, K. S., Cheong, H. K., Kim, E. A., Kim, K. R., Oh, B. H. & Hong, C. H. (2009). Nutritional Risk and Cognitive Impairment in the Elderly. *Archives of Gerontology and Geriatrics*, 48 (1), 95–99. https://doi.org/10.1016/j.archger.2007.11.001.

Leslie, W. & Hankey, C. (2015). Aging, Nutritional Status, and Health. *Healthcare*, 3 (3), 648–58. https://doi.org/10.3390/healthcare3030648.

Lesourd, B. (2004). Nutrition: A Major Factor Influencing Immunity in the Elderly. *The Journal of Nutrition, Health & Aging*, 8 (1), 28–37.

Lesourd, B. (2006). Nutritional Factors and Immunological Ageing. *The Proceedings of the Nutrition Society*, 65 (3), 319–25.

Lin, P. H., Sermersheim, M., Li, M., Lee, P. H. U., Steinberg, S. M. & Ma, J. (2017). Zinc in Wound Healing Modulation. *Nutrients*, 10 (1). https://doi.org/10.3390/nu10010016.

Malara, A., Sgrò, G., Caruso, C., Ceravolo, F., Curinga, G., Renda, G. F., Spadea, F., Garo, M. & Rispoli, V. (2014). Relationship between Cognitive Impairment and Nutritional Assessment on Functional Status in Calabrian Long-Term-Care. *Clinical Interventions in Aging*, 9, 105–10. https://doi.org/10.2147/CIA.S54611.

Mamta, B., Priya, S., Rachna, K. & Manjula, S. (2018). A Pilot Study on Prevalence of Malnutrition, Pain, Depression and Anxiety in Elderly Population in Delhi. *Journal of Clinical Gerontology and Geriatrics*, 9, 91–98. https://doi.org/10.24816/jcgg.2018.v9i3.04.

Martone, A. M., Onder, G., Vetrano, D. L., Ortolani, E., Tosato, M., Marzetti, E. & Landi, F. (2013). Anorexia of Aging: A Modifiable Risk Factor for Frailty. *Nutrients*, 5 (10), 4126–33. https://doi.org/10.3390/nu5104126.

Naidoo, U. (2016). Nutritional Strategies to Ease Anxiety. Harvard Health Blog. April 13, 2016. https://www.health.harvard.edu/blog/nutritional-strategies-to-ease-anxiety-201604139441.

Megabiaw, B. & Rahman, A. (2013). Prevalence and determinants of chronic malnutrition among under-5 children in Ethiopia. *International Journal of Child Health and Nutrition*, 3 (2), 230-6. https://doi.org/10.6000/1929-4247.2013.02.03.5.

Meijers, J. M., Halfens, R. J., Neyens, J. C., Luiking, Y. C., Verlaan, G. & Schols, J. M. (2012). Predicting Falls in Elderly Receiving Home Care: The Role of Malnutrition and Impaired Mobility. *The Journal of Nutrition, Health & Aging*, 16 (7), 654–58.

Messaoudi, M., Lalonde, R., Violle, N., Javelot, H., Desor, D., Nejdi, A., Bisson, J., et al. (2011). Assessment of Psychotropic-like Properties of a Probiotic Formulation (Lactobacillus Helveticus R0052 and Bifidobacterium Longum R0175) in Rats and Human Subjects. *The British Journal of Nutrition*, 105 (5), 755–64. https://doi.org/10.1017/S0007114510004319.

Miu, K. Y., Chan, C. W., Lam, P. S., Kok, C., Lam, K. Y. & Kwok, S. L. (2018). Differences in Risk Factors among Early and Late Readmission of Elderly Patients from Convalescence Care Unit and 30 and 90 Days Outcome: A Cohort Study. *Aging Medicine and Healthcare (Journal of Clinical Gerontology & Geriatrics)*, 9 (4), 137–42. https://doi.org/10.33879/JCGG.2018.1801.

Mokhber, N., Majdi, M., Ali-Abadi, M., Shakeri, M., Kimiagar, M., Salek, R., Moghaddam, P. A., et al. (2011). Association between Malnutrition and Depression in Elderly People in Razavi Khorasan: A Population Based-Study in Iran. *Iranian Journal of Public Health*, 40 (2), 67–74.

Molnar, J. A., Underdown, M. J. & Clark, W. A. (2014). Nutrition and Chronic Wounds. *Advances in Wound Care*, 3 (11), 663–81. https://doi.org/10.1089/wound.2014.0530.

Morley, J. E. & Kraenzle, D. (1994). Causes of Weight Loss in a Community Nursing Home. *Journal of the American Geriatrics Society*, 42 (6), 583–85.

Morley, J. E., Kumar, V. B., Mattammal, M. B., Farr, S., Morley, P. M. K. & Flood, J. F. (1996). Inhibition of Feeding by a Nitric Oxide Synthase Inhibitor: Effects of Aging. *European Journal of Pharmacology*, 311 (1), 15–9. https://doi.org/10.1016/0014-2999(96)00546-8.

Moss, C., Dhillo, W. S., Frost, G. & Hickson, M. (2012). Gastrointestinal Hormones: The Regulation of Appetite and the Anorexia of Ageing. *Journal of Human Nutrition and Dietetics: The Official Journal of the British Dietetic Association*, 25 (1), 3–15. https://doi.org/10.1111/j.1365-277X.2011.01211.x.

Muscaritoli, M., Anker, S. D., Argilés, J., Aversa, Z., Bauer, J. M., Biolo, G., Boirie, Y., et al. (2010). Consensus Definition of Sarcopenia, Cachexia and Pre-Cachexia: Joint Document Elaborated by Special Interest Groups (SIG) 'Cachexia-Anorexia in Chronic Wasting Diseases' and 'Nutrition in Geriatrics. *Clinical Nutrition (Edinburgh, Scotland)*, 29 (2), 154–9. https://doi.org/10.1016/j.clnu.2009.12.004.

Natarajan, V. S., Ravindran, S., Sivashanmugam., Thyagarajan., Kailash, K., Krishnaswamy, B., Suresh, B. & Prabhu, P. (1993). Assessment of Nutrient Intake and Associated Factors in an Indian Elderly

Population. *Age and Ageing*, 22 (2), 103–8. https://doi.org/10.1093/ageing/22.2.103.

Haesler, E. (2014). National Pressure Ulcer Advisory Panel (U.S.), European Pressure Ulcer Advisory Panel, and Pan Pacific Pressure Injury Alliance. *Prevention and Treatment of Pressure Ulcers.*

Nazan, S. & Buket, K. (2018). Evaluation of Nutritional Status of Elderly Patients Presenting to the Family Health Center. *Pakistan Journal of Medical Sciences*, 34 (2), 446–51. https://doi.org/10.12669/pjms.342.14936.

Neyens, J., Halfens, R., Spreeuwenberg, M., Meijers, J., Luiking, Y., Verlaan, G. & Schols, J. (2013). Malnutrition Is Associated with an Increased Risk of Falls and Impaired Activity in Elderly Patients in Dutch Residential Long-Term Care (LTC): A Cross-Sectional Study. *Archives of Gerontology and Geriatrics*, 56 (1), 265–69. https://doi.org/10.1016/j.archger.2012.08.005.

Orrevall, Y., Tishelman, C., Permert, J. & Cederholm, T. (2009). Nutritional Support and Risk Status among Cancer Patients in Palliative Home Care Services. *Supportive Care in Cancer: Official Journal of the Multinational Association of Supportive Care in Cancer*, 17 (2), 153–61. https://doi.org/10.1007/s00520-008-0467-4.

Pirlich, M. & Lochs, H. (2001). Nutrition in the Elderly. *Best Practice & Research. Clinical Gastroenterology*, 15 (6), 869–84. https://doi.org/10.1053/bega.2001.0246.

Posthauer, M., Banks, M., Dorner, B. & Schols, J. M. G. (2015). The Role of Nutrition for Pressure Ulcer Management: National Pressure Ulcer Advisory Panel, European Pressure Ulcer Advisory Panel, and Pan Pacific Pressure Injury Alliance White Paper. *Advances in Skin & Wound Care*, 28 (4), 175–88. https://doi.org/10.1097/01.ASW.0000461911.31139.62.

Prell, T. & Perner, C. (2018). Disease Specific Aspects of Malnutrition in Neurogeriatric Patients. *Frontiers in Aging Neuroscience*, 10, 80. https://doi.org/10.3389/fnagi.2018.00080.

Prentice, A. (2004). Diet, Nutrition and the Prevention of Osteoporosis. *Public Health Nutrition*, 7 (1A), 227–43.

Rahman, A. & Chowdhury, S. (2007). Determinants of chronic malnutrition among preschool children in Bangladesh. *Journal of Biosocial Science*, 39 (2), 161-173. https://doi.org/10.1017/S0021932006001295.

Rahman, A. & Biswas, C. S. (2009). Nutritional status of under-5 children in Bangladesh. *South Asian Journal of Population and Health*, 2 (1), 1-11.

Rahman, A. & Harding, A. (2011). Social and health costs of tobacco smoking in Australia: level, trend and determinants. *International Journal of Statistics and Systems*, 6 (4), 399-411.

Rahman, A. & Harding, A. (2013). Prevalence of overweight and obesity epidemic in Australia: some causes and consequences. *JP Journal of Biostatistics*, 10 (1), 31-48.

Rahman, A. & Sapkota, M. (2014). Knowledge on vitamin A rich foods among mothers of preschool children in Nepal: Impacts on public health and policy concerns. *Science Journal of Public Health*, 2 (4), 316-22. https://doi.org/10.11648/j.sjph.20140204.22.

Rahman, A. (2016). Significant risk factors for childhood malnutrition: Evidence from an Asian developing country. *Science Journal of Public Health*, 4 (1), 16-27.

Rahman, A., Chowdury, S., Karim, A. & Ahmed, S. (2008). Factors associated with nutritional status of children in Bangladesh: A multivariate analysis. *Demography India: population-society-economy-environment-interactions*, 37 (1), 95-109.

Rahman, A., Chowdhury, S. & Hossain, D. (2009). Acute malnutrition in Bangladeshi children's levels and determinants. *Asia-Pacific Journal of Public Health*, 21 (3), 294-302. https://doi.org/ 10.1177/1010539509335399.

Rahman, A. & Hakim, M. A. (2016). Measuring modified mass-energy equivalence in nutritional epidemiology: A proposal to adapt the biophysical modeling approach. *International Journal of Statistics in Medical Research*, 5 (3), 219-223.

Rahman, A., Hakim, M. A., Hanif, M. A., Islam, M. R. & Kamruzzaman, M. (2016). Dietary practices, health status and hygiene observance of slum kids: A pilot study in an Asian developing country. *JP Journal of Biostatistics*, 13 (2), 195-208. https://doi.org/10.17654/BO013020195.

Rahman, A. (2017). Estimating small area health-related characteristics of populations: A methodological review. *Geospatial Health*, 12 (1), 3-14. https://doi.org/10.4081/gh.2017.495.

Rahman, A. & Rahman, M. S. (2019). Rural-urban differentials of childhood malnutrition in Bangladesh. *International Journal of Child Health and Nutrition*, 35-42. https://doi.org/10.6000/1929-4247.2019.08.01.5.

Rahman, A. (2019).Geospatial, socioeconomic, demographic and health determinants of childhood mortality in Bangladesh. *Demography India: population-society-economy-environment-interactions*, 48 (2), 74-85.

Rahman, A., Rahman, M. S. & Rahman, M. A. (2019). Determinants of infant mortality in Bangladesh: A nationally surveyed data analysis. *International Journal of Child Health and Nutrition*, 8 (3), 93-102. https://doi.org/10.6000/1929-4247.2019.08.03.3.

Rajkamal, R., Singh, J., Stalin, P. & Muthurajesh, E. (2015). Prevalence and Determinants of Overweight and Obesity among Elderly Population in an Urban Area of Puducherry. *International Journal of Medical Science and Public Health*, 4 (3), 369. https://doi.org/10.5455/ijmsph.2015.3110201477.

Ranganath, L., Sedgwick, I., Morgan, L., Wright, J. & Marks, V. (1998). The Ageing Entero-Insular Axis. *Diabetologia*, 41 (11), 1309–13. https://doi.org/10.1007/s001250051070.

Rasheed, S. & Woods, R. T. (2013). Malnutrition and Quality of Life in Older People: A Systematic Review and Meta-Analysis. *Ageing Research Reviews*, 12 (2), 561–66. https://doi.org/10.1016/j.arr.2012.11.003.

Ratnaprabha, G. K., Farah, N. F., Twinkle, A., Naveen, J. T. & Ashit, B. X. (2015). Prevalence of Obesity and its Associated Factors among Elderly in a Rural Area of South Karnataka. *Annals of Community Health*, 2 (3), 15-21.

Rizzoli, R. & Bonjour, J. P. (1999). Malnutrition and osteoporosis. *Z Gerontol Geriat,* 32, Suppl. 1, I/31–I/37.

Rodríguez-Tadeo, A., Wall-Medrano, A., Gaytan-Vidaña, M. E., Campos, A., Ornelas-Contreras, M. & Novelo-Huerta, H. I. (2012). Malnutrition Risk Factors among the Elderly from the US-Mexico Border: The 'One Thousand' Study. *The Journal of Nutrition, Health & Aging*, 16 (5), 426–31.

Rubenstein, L. Z., Harker, J. O., Salvà, A., Guigoz, Y. & Vellas, B. (2001). Screening for Undernutrition in Geriatric Practice: Developing the Short-Form Mini-Nutritional Assessment (MNA-SF). *The Journals of Gerontology. Series A, Biological Sciences and Medical Sciences*, 56 (6), M366-372. https://doi.org/10.1093/gerona/56.6.m366.

Saka, B., Kaya, O., Ozturk, G. B., Erten, N. & Karan, M. A. (2010). Malnutrition in the Elderly and Its Relationship with Other Geriatric Syndromes. *Clinical Nutrition (Edinburgh, Scotland)*, 29 (6), 745–48. https://doi.org/10.1016/j.clnu.2010.04.006.

Salazar, N, Valdés-Varela, L., González, S., Gueimonde, M. & de Los Reyes-Gavilán, C. G. (2017). Nutrition and the Gut Microbiome in the Elderly. *Gut Microbes*, 8 (2), 82–97. https://doi.org/10.1080/19490976.2016.1256525.

Saletti, A., Lindgren, E. Y., Johansson, L. & Cederholm, T. (2000). Nutritional Status According to Mini Nutritional Assessment in an Institutionalized Elderly Population in Sweden. *Gerontology*, 46 (3), 139–45. https://doi.org/10.1159/000022149.

Schiffman, S. S. (1993). Perception of Taste and Smell in Elderly Persons. *Critical Reviews in Food Science and Nutrition*, 33 (1), 17–26. https://doi.org/10.1080/10408399309527608.

Shankar, R. & Balamurugan, S. S. (2011). Prevalence of Chronic Energy Deficiency, Overweight and Obesity Among the Geriatric Population in the Rural Area in Tamilnadu. *Sri Ramachandra Journal of Medicine*, 4, 24-29.

Siddique, N., O'Donoghue, M., Casey, M. C. & Walsh, J. B. (2017). Malnutrition in the Elderly and Its Effects on Bone Health - A Review.

Clinical Nutrition ESPEN, 21, 31–39. https://doi.org/10.1016/j.clnesp.2017.06.001.

Silva, P. B., Trindade, L. C. T., Gallucci, M. C. & Schirr, R. A. (2013). Prevalence of Malnutrition and Pain in Patients Admitted by the Screening Service of an Oncologic Hospital. *RevistaDor*, 14 (4), 263–66. https://doi.org/10.1590/S1806-00132013000400006.

Singh, D. K. A., Manaf, Z. A., Yusoff, N. A. M., Muhammad, N. A., Phan, M.F. & Shahar, S. (2014). Correlation between Nutritional Status and Comprehensive Physical Performance Measures among Older Adults with Undernourishment in Residential Institutions. *Clinical Interventions in Aging*, 9, 1415–23. https://doi.org/10.2147/CIA.S64997.

Smoliner, C., Kristina N., Wagner, K., Hartig, W., Lochs, H. & Pirlich, M. (2009). Malnutrition and Depression in the Institutionalised Elderly. *The British Journal of Nutrition*, 102 (11), 1663–67. https://doi.org/10.1017/S0007114509990900.

Söderström, L., Adolfsson, E. T., Rosenblad, A., Frid, H., Saletti, A. & Bergkvist, L. (2013). Mealtime Habits and Meal Provision Are Associated with Malnutrition among Elderly Patients Admitted to Hospital. *Clinical Nutrition (Edinburgh, Scotland)*, 32 (2), 281–88. https://doi.org/10.1016/j.clnu.2012.07.013.

Stuck, A. E., Walthert, J. M., Nikolaus, T., Büla, C. J., Hohmann, C. & Beck, J. C. (1999). Risk Factors for Functional Status Decline in Community-Living Elderly People: A Systematic Literature Review. *Social Science & Medicine*, 48 (4), 445–69.

Suominen, M., Muurinen, S., Routasalo, P., Soini, H., Suur-Uski, I., Peiponen, A., Finne-Soveri, H. & Pitkala, K. H. (2005). Malnutrition and Associated Factors among Aged Residents in All Nursing Homes in Helsinki. *European Journal of Clinical Nutrition*, 59 (4), 578–83. https://doi.org/10.1038/sj.ejcn.1602111.

Swami, H. M., Bhatia, V., Gupta, V. K. & Bhatia, S. P. S. (2005). An Epidemiological Study of Obesity Among Elderly in Chandigarh. *Indian Journal of Community Medicine*, 30 (1), 11-13.

Takahashi, H., Chiba, T., Tairabune, T., Kimura, Y., Wakabayashi, G., Takahashi, K. & Kudo, K. (2014). A Retrospective Study on the Influence of Nutritional Status on Pain Management in Cancer Patients Using the Transdermal Fentanyl Patch. *Biological & Pharmaceutical Bulletin*, 37 (5), 853–57.

Tamura, B. K., Bell, C. L., Masaki, K. H. & Amella, E. J. (2013). Factors Associated with Weight Loss, Low BMI, and Malnutrition among Nursing Home Patients: A Systematic Review of the Literature. *Journal of the American Medical Directors Association*, 14 (9), 649–55. https://doi.org/10.1016/j.jamda.2013.02.022.

Tseng, B. S., Marsh, D. R., Hamilton, M. T. & Booth, F. W. (1995). Strength and Aerobic Training Attenuate Muscle Wasting and Improve Resistance to the Development of Disability with Aging. *The Journals of Gerontology. Series A, Biological Sciences and Medical Sciences*, 50, 113–19. https://doi.org/10.1093/gerona/50a.special_issue.113.

Vanderwee, K., Clays, E., Bocquaert, L., Gobert, M., Folens, B. & Defloor, T. (2010). Malnutrition and Associated Factors in Elderly Hospital Patients: A Belgian Cross-Sectional, Multi-Centre Study. *Clinical Nutrition (Edinburgh, Scotland)*, 29 (4), 469–76. https://doi.org/10.1016/j.clnu.2009.12.013.

Vandewoude, M., Carolyn, F. J., Alish, J., Sauer, A. C. & Hegazi, R. A. (2012). Malnutrition-Sarcopenia Syndrome: Is This the Future of Nutrition Screening and Assessment for Older Adults? *Journal of Aging Research*, 651570. https://doi.org/10.1155/2012/651570.

Vassilakou, T., Triantafillou, G. & Evrenoglou, L. (2017). Early Identification of Malnutrition Risk Among Free-Living Elderly Persons in Athens, Greece. *The Journal of Aging Research and Clinical Practice*, 6, 193-99. http://dx.doi.org/10.14283/jarcp.2017.26.

Vedantam, A., Subramanian, V., Rao, N. V. & John, K. R. (2010). Malnutrition in Free-Living Elderly in Rural South India: Prevalence and Risk Factors. *Public Health Nutrition*, 13 (9), 1328–32. https://doi.org/10.1017/S1368980009991674.

Vellas, B., Lauque, S., Andrieu, S., Nourhashemi, F., Rolland, Y., Baumgartner, Y. & Garry, P. (2001). Nutrition Assessment in the

Elderly. *Current Opinion in Clinical Nutrition and Metabolic Care*, 4 (1), 5–8.

Vivanti, A., Ward, N. & Haines, T. (2011). Nutritional Status and Associations with Falls, Balance, Mobility, and Functionality during Hospital Admission. *The Journal of Nutrition, Health & Aging*, 15 (5), 388–91.

Wada, H. (2000). Problems and Strategies in the Treatment of Mental Disorders in Elderly Patients with Physical Illness. *Nihon Ronen Igakkai Zasshi. Japanese Journal of Geriatrics*, 37 (11), 885–88.

Wei, J. M., Li, S., Claytor, L., Partridge, J. & Goates, S. (2018). Prevalence and Predictors of Malnutrition in Elderly Chinese Adults: Results from the China Health and Retirement Longitudinal Study. *Public Health Nutrition*, 21 (17), 1-6. doi: 10.1017/S1368980018002227.

Wei, K., Nyunt, M., Gao, Q., Wee, S. L. & Ng, T. (2017). Frailty and Malnutrition: Related and Distinct Syndrome Prevalence and Association among Community-Dwelling Older Adults: Singapore Longitudinal Ageing Studies. *Journal of the American Medical Directors Association*, 18 (12), 1019–28. https://doi.org/10.1016/j.jamda.2017.06.017.

Wei, K., Nyunt, M., Gao, Q., Wee, S., Yap, K. & Ng, T. (2018). Association of Frailty and Malnutrition with Long-Term Functional and Mortality Outcomes among Community-Dwelling Older Adults: Results from the Singapore Longitudinal Aging Study 1. *JAMA Network Open*, 1 (3), e180650. https://doi.org/10.1001/jamanetworkopen.2018.0650.

WHO | The World Health Report 2004 - Changing History. n.d. WHO. Accessed June 6, 2019. https://www.who.int/whr/2004/en/.

WHO | The World Health Report 2008 - Primary Health Care (Now More Than Ever). n.d. WHO. Accessed June 6, 2019. https://www.who.int/whr/2008/en/.

Wojszel, Z. B. (2006). Determinants of Nutritional Status of Older People in Long-Term Care Settings on the Example of the Nursing Home in Białystok. *Advances in Medical Sciences*, 51, 168–73.

Wolfe, W. S., Frongillo, E. A. & Valois, P. (2003). Understanding the Experience of Food Insecurity by Elders Suggests Ways to Improve Its Measurement. *The Journal of Nutrition*, 133 (9), 2762–69. https://doi.org/10.1093/jn/133.9.2762.

World Population Prospects. Accessed June 6, 2019. https://population.un.org/wpp/Publications/Files/WPP2012_HIGHLIGHTS.pdf.

Yeh, S. S. & Schuster, M. W. (1999). Geriatric Cachexia: The Role of Cytokines. *The American Journal of Clinical Nutrition*, 70 (2), 183–97. https://doi.org/10.1093/ajcn.70.2.183.

Yoshimura, K., Yamada, M., Kajiwara, Y., Nishiguchi, S. & Aoyama, T. (2013). Relationship between Depression and Risk of Malnutrition among Community-Dwelling Young-Old and Old-Old Elderly People. *Aging & Mental Health*, 17 (4), 456–60. https://doi.org/10.1080/13607863.2012.743961.

Zeanandin, G., Molato, O., Le Duff, F., Guérin, O., Hébuterne, X. & Schneider, S. M. (2012). Impact of Restrictive Diets on the Risk of Undernutrition in a Free-Living Elderly Population. *Clinical Nutrition (Edinburgh, Scotland)*, 31 (1), 69–73. https://doi.org/10.1016/j.clnu.2011.08.007.

In: Malnutrition
Editor: Azizur Rahman
ISBN: 978-1-53617-597-4

Chapter 2

PREVALENCE OF MALNUTRITION AMONG RURAL BENGALEE CHILDREN OF HOOGHLY DISTRICT, WEST BENGAL, INDIA

Soma Pal* and Kaushik Bose, PhD
Department of Anthropology, Vidyasagar University,
Midnapore, West Bengal, India

ABSTRACT

Child undernutrition remains an enduring public health concern in low-income and middle-income countries. The present cross-sectional study was undertaken to assess the prevalence of malnutrition among rural primary school children utilizing new internationally accepted age and sex specific cut offs of body mass index (BMI). Our study was conducted among 822 rural primary school children of Jangipara Block of Hooghly District, West Bengal, India. A total of 812 children (431 girls; 381 boys) aged from 6 to 10 years were eligible for the present study. Anthropometric variables like height in cm and weight in kg were measured according to standard procedures. The BMI was computed

*Corresponding Author's Email: palsoma05@gmail.com.

following the standard equation to evaluate the nutritional status of these children. All data was analysed in Statistical Package for Social Sciences (SPSS, version 16.0) software and significance level was set at $p<0.05$. Results of Independent Sample t test revealed that there was no statistically significant sex difference in mean height, weight and BMI. Significant age differences were observed for girls (HT: $F = 117.597$, $p<0.001$; WT: $F = 37.210$, $p<0.001$; and BMI: $F = 3.988$, $p<0.01$) as well as boys (HT: $F = 104.184$, $p<0.001$; WT: $F = 26.602$, $p<0.001$ and BMI: $F = 2.838$, $p<0.05$). The prevalence of overall thinness, normal, overweight and obese was 48.5%, 45.4%, 4.8% and 1.2%, respectively. No significant age group and sex wise differences were observed in prevalence of different nutritional status category except in overweight ($\chi^2 = 9.538$, df = 4 and $p<0.05$) category. Results of χ^2 test also revealed that age combined sex differences in different grades of nutritional status were not statistically significant ($\chi^2 = 4.112$; df = 5 and $p>0.05$). Results indicated that girls were thinner than boys. In contrast, boys were prone to be overweight and obese. All regional studies (including the present) had reported very high prevalence rate of overall thinness according to World Health Organization. Most of the international and national studies had observed a lower rate of overall thinness than our study. In conclusion, the present study clearly indicated that half of the studied girls (50.6%) were undernourished and more boys were overweight and obese. Surveillance of present nutritional schemes and state specific appropriate and immediate new nutritional interventions are required to ameliorate the problem of malnutrition.

Keywords: malnutrition, children, nutritional status, thinness, body mass index

INTRODUCTION

Malnutrition is an abnormal physiological condition caused by inadequate, imbalanced or excessive consumption of the macronutrients (carbohydrates, protein and fats) that provide dietary energy and the micronutrients (vitamins and minerals) that are essential for physical and cognitive growth and development. In many developing countries under-nutrition (Rahman et al., 2008) and over-nutrition are occurring simultaneously among different population groups, a phenomenon referred to as the *"double burden"* of malnutrition. The consequence of malnutrition is poor infant and child growth and an excess of morbidity and mortality in adults and children alike (Rahman and Chowdhury, 2007; Rahman, 2016). It includes all deviations from adequate nutrition including undernutrition (a deficiency of proteins, carbohydrates and fats and/or vitamins and minerals) and overnutrition (an excess of certain food components such as saturated fats and added sugars in combination with low physical activity), and specific deficiencies (or excesses) of essential nutrients such as vitamins and minerals. Now-a-days, many developing countries are experiencing undernutrition and over-nutrition among different population groups, a condition referred to as *"double burden"* of malnutrition (FAO, 2011; Hakim and Rahman, 2016). It is considered to be a major public health concern that causes several ill-health conditions, premature mortality and morbidities (Nandy et al., 2005; Black et al., 2008; Rahman et al., 2009). The health consequences of prolonged state of malnutrition among children and adolescents include delayed physical growth and impaired motor and cognitive development, diminished cognitive performance, lower Intellectual Quotient (IQ) levels, poor psychosocial development, greater behavioural problems and reduced adult size leading to decreased economic productivity (Park, 2005; Mengisty et al., 2013; Rahman and Biswas, 2009; Megabiaw and Rahman, 2013; Rahman and Rahman, 2019; Rahman, 2019).

In low-income and middle-income countries, maternal and child undernutrition remains an enduring public health concern (Black et al., 2008; Rahman et al., 2016; Rahman and Hakim, 2016a). Black et al., (2013) estimated that undernutrition including fetal growth restriction, stunting, wasting, and deficiencies of vitamin A and zinc along with suboptimum breastfeeding attributed to the cause of 3·1 million child deaths annually or 45% of all child deaths in 2011. Similar findings have been revealed by some other researchers conducted studies in other countries including Bangladesh (Rahman and Hakim, 2016b, c; Rahman and Sapkota, 2014; Rahman et al., 2019). Beyond the very high social cost (Rahman and Harding, 2011, 2013; Rahman 2017), the estimated cost to the global economy caused by malnutrition, as a result of lost productivity and direct health care costs, could account for as much as 5 percent of global gross domestic product (GDP), equivalent to US$3.5 trillion per year or US$500 per person. The estimated costs of undernutrition and micronutrient deficiencies are equivalent to US$1.4–2.1 trillion per year or 2–3 percent of global GDP. While in 2012, the cumulative cost of all non-communicable diseases (NCD), for which overweight and obesity are leading risk factors, were estimated to be about US$1.4 trillion (Food and Agricultural Organization, 2013).

Anthropometric method has been used during childhood and adolescence in many contexts related to nutritional status. Nutritional status of children has been traditionally assessed by utilizing anthropometric measurements of height, weight, mid upper arm circumference (MUAC) and skinfold thickness (e.g., biceps, triceps, subscapular and suprailliac). Anthropometric measures have been widely used because of its simplicity, reliable, non-invasive, portable, inexpensive and universally accepted technique to assess child undernutrition (WHO, 1995). The most commonly used conventional anthropometric measures of undernutrition among children such as stunting (low height-for-age), underweight (low weight-for-age), wasting (low weight-for-age), and thinness (low BMI-for-age) (WHO, 1995; Nandy et al., 2005; and Mondal and Sen, 2010; Rahman and Chowdhury, 2007). In India, several studies (both nationally representative study and independent researcher) were undertaken among children under five years to assess the magnitude of undernutrition using conventional indices. The National Family Health Survey-4 (NFHS-4 was conducted during 2015-16) data reported 38.4% under five years children have stunted growth, 21.0% children under five years are suffering from wasting and 35.7% under five years children have low weight for age (underweight). West Bengal State has 28.5% stunted, 16.7% wasted (6.0% severely wasted) and 26.2% underweight children under five years as per NFHS-4 (IIPS).

Recently, new international age and sex-specific cut offs of BMI for the age range of 2-18 years have been developed by Cole et al., to define child overweight and obesity in 2000 and thinness in 2007. In the later study, undernutrition has been termed as thinness defined as low BMI for age and it has been graded as III, II, I (severe, moderate and mild, respectively) similar to adult chronic energy deficiency (CED) grades ofIII, II and I (Cole et al., 2007). Worldwide, several researchers (da Silva et al., 2008; Bovet et al., 2011; Ene-Obong et al., 2012; Caleyachetty et al., 2012; Rana et al., 2012; Mustaq et al., 2012; Ejike et al., 2013; Wamba et al., 2013; Akinpelu et al., 2014; Schonbeck et al., 2014; O'Dea et al., 2014; Zhang et al., 2016; Partap et al., 2017) carried out their studies among children and adolescents to assess the prevalence of thinness utilizing BMI cut-offs according to Cole et al., (2007). Numerous researchers have conducted investigations among urban children (Bansal and Joshi, 2013; Hasan et al., 2016; Das et al., 2017; Chudasama et al., 2017; Rahman et al., 2019) as well as tribal children (Sikdar, 2012; Singh and Mondal, 2013; Longkumar, 2013; Singh et al., 2014; Mondal et al., 2015; Singh et al., 2015; Das et al., 2016; Bharthi et al., 2017; and Bartwal, 2017) from different states of India to assess the nutritional status of the children using same cut-offs (Cole et al., 2007). Several previous studies have also been undertaken to assess the prevalence rate of thinness among rural children [Chakraborty and Bose, 2009; Mondal and Sen, 2010; Mondal et al., 2011; Das et al., 2012b; Das et al., 2015; Das et al., 2017a; Das et al., 2017b; Debnath et al., 2018 and Pal and Bose (communicated)], children of semi-urban area (Banik and Chatterjee, 2010) as well as tribal children (Bisai et al., 2010; Das and Bose, 2011a; Das and Bose, 2011b; Das et al., 2012a; and Mandal and Bose, 2014) from different districts of West Bengal state utilizing the internationally accepted BMI cut offs developed by Cole et al., (2007). Nevertheless, limited studies have been carried out among under five years children (Mandal et al., 2009) and children of childhood age group [Mandal and Bose, 2014 and Pal and Bose (communicated)] of Hooghly District, West Bengal State of India for assessing thinness utilizing same international age and sex specific BMI cut offs proposed by Cole et al., (2007). In view of the above, the present investigation was undertaken among children aged 6 to 10 years old of Hooghly District, West Bengal, India to assess the prevalence of malnutrition utilizing international age and sex specific BMI cut offs proposed by Cole et al., (2000 and 2007).

MATERIALS AND METHODS

Study Area and People

Our cross-sectional study was undertaken among primary school children of Jangipara Block of Hooghly District, West Bengal, India. Jangipara is located 45 kilometres away from Chinsurah, the headquarters of Hooghly District or around 45 kilometres away from Kolkata, the capital of West Bengal. Study participants were selected from eleven Government aided primary schools of Jangipara Block (ten schools from Mundalika Gram Panchayet and one school from Kotalpur Gram Panchayet) of Hooghly District. Gram Panchayet is the village level governing authority. Mundalika Gram Panchayet and Kotalpur Gram Panchayet were purposively selected for the convenience of conducting fieldwork. Schools were chosen by opportunity sampling on basis of easy accessibility of road connectivity to the schools and convenience of data collection. All students of both sexes from 6 to 10 years old were eligible for this study. Students from 1st standard to 4th standard were selected for this investigation because of the inclusion criterion of this study. All children were Bengalees. Necessary approval was obtained from the higher school authorities before the commencement of data collection. Objectives of the study were explained clearly to the Head Teacher of the schools prior to the collection of data. The present study was carried out in accordance with the ethical guidelines for human experiments, as laid down by the Helsinki Declaration of 2000 (Touitou et al., 2004).

Sample and Sample Size

The sample size was determined by using the standard formula ($n = z^2pq/d^2$) according to Naing et al., (2006) where $z = 1.96$ (95% Confidence Interval), p = prevalence, $q = (1-p)$, and d = precision. The minimum estimated sample size was 756 [$(1.96^2 \times 0.77 \times 0.23)/0.03^2$]. The minimum sample size was estimated based on 77.0% prevalence (p) of thinness among rural children of Paschim Medinipur (Das et al., 2012b) with desired precision (d) of 3%, where q = (1 - 0.77) and z = 1.96. A total of 822 children were measured and interviewed by with structured schedules. Out of 822 children, 6 children were excluded from the study because of inappropriate age group i.e., children aged less than 6 years and above 10 years and 4 children were also excluded for missing of date of birth. Hence, the final sample size for the present investigation was 812 children (girls 431; boys 381) aged from 6 to 10 years.

Anthropometric Measurements and Assessment of Nutritional Status

Anthropometric variables such as height (cm.) and weight (kg.) were measured by following standard procedures according to Lohman et al., (1988). The Body Mass Index (BMI, kg/m^2) was calculated as weight/height^2 (kg/m^2). Date of birth of children was collected from the admission register of the school. Hence, actual age of the child was calculated by deducting the date of birth from date of survey. Children were measured and interviewed at their respective schools using structured schedule. All data were collected by the first author (SP) during November, 2017 to September, 2018. Technical errors of measurements (TEM) were calculated and were found to be within acceptable limits (Ulijaszek and Kerr, 1999).

The prevalence of malnutrition (in terms of thinness, overweight and obesity) or nutritional status of present studied children was evaluated by utilizing age and sex specific cut-off points of BMI as described by Cole et al., (2000 and 2007). The cut off values of BMI are presented in Table 1. These internationally accepted references have been suggested to encourage direct comparison of childhood thinness and overweight-obesity that provide a classification for the worldwide public health purposes (Cole et al., 2000 and 2007).

Table 1. Age and sex specific international cut-off values for assessing thinness, overweight and obese among children (based on Cole et al., 2007 & 2000)

Age (Yrs.)	BOYS					
	Thinness Grade III	**Thinness Grade II**	**Thinness Grade I**	**Normal**	**Overweight**	**Obese**
6.5	12.45	13.10	14.04	14.04 – 17.71	17.71	20.23
7.5	12.41	13.09	14.08	14.08 – 18.16	18.16	21.09
8.5	12.45	13.17	14.24	14.24 – 18.76	18.76	22.17
9.5	12.57	13.24	14.49	14.49 – 19.46	19.46	23.39
10.5	12.77	13.58	14.80	14.80 – 20.20	20.20	24.57
	GIRLS					
6.5	12.28	12.90	13.82	13.82 – 17.53	17.53	20.08
7.5	12.27	12.95	13.93	13.93 – 18.03	18.03	21.01
8.5	12.37	13.08	14.14	14.14 – 18.69	18.69	22.18
9.5	12.53	13.29	14.43	14.43 – 19.45	19.45	23.46
10.5	12.78	13.59	14.81	14.81 – 20.29	20.29	27.77

Mid-year of ages of the children is considered for present analysis.

Statistical Analysis

The data was analysed using Statistical Package for Social Sciences (SPSS, version 16.0). Independent sample t-tests were performed to observe the age specific sex differences in anthropometric variables. One-way ANOVA (F test) tests were done to see significant age variations in mean anthropometric values for both sexes. Chi-square (χ^2) analysis was done to assess the age group and sex specific differences in prevalence of different nutritional status category. Chi-square (χ^2) test was also performed to see the age combined sex differences in BMI based nutritional status. The Yates correction term was also considered. This correction terms adds to the accuracy of the χ^2 analysis determinants when the number of cases is small (<5 cases) in any cell. Statistical significance level was set at the $p<0.05$.

RESULTS

Table 2 represents the descriptive statistics (mean and standard deviation), t test and One-Way ANOVA (F) test value of anthropometric variables namely height, weight and BMI. Results of t test indicated that there were no significant sex differences in mean height, weight and BMI. The results of F test revealed that significant age differences existed in mean height, weight and BMI for girls (HT: $F = 117.597$, $p<0.001$; WT: $F = 37.210$, $p<0.001$; and BMI: $F = 3.988$, $p<0.01$) as well as boys (HT: $F = 104.184$, $p<0.001$; WT: $F = 26.602$, $p<0.001$ and BMI: $F = 2.838$, $p<0.05$).

Table 2. Descriptive statistics (Mean & SD), t and F value of the anthropometric variables

Variable	Sex	Age (Years)					F (p)
		6	7	8	9	10	
Height (cm.)	G	113.1(4.9)	116.3(5.7)	122.3(5.4)	127.1(5.6)	131.6(7.5)	117.597***
	B	112.7(5.8)	117.5(5.7)	123.2(4.2)	127.9(6.4)	130.6(6.1)	104.184***
	t	0.465	-1.412	-1.412	-0.870	0.7222	
Weight (kg.)	G	18.1(3.4)	19.5(4.4)	22.1(4.4)	24.1(5.2)	27.1(6.1)	37.210***
	B	18.5(4.1)	20.0(3.4)	22.9(4.3)	25.4(6.5)	25.4(6.0)	26.602***
	t	-0.548	-0.784	-1.363	-1.622	1.426	
BMI (kg/m2)	G	14.0(1.7)	14.3(2.1)	14.7(2.1)	14.8(2.4)	15.5(2.3)	3.988**
	B	14.5(2.2)	14.4(1.5)	15.0(2.2)	15.4(3.1)	14.8(2.4)	2.838*
	t	-1.115	-0.331	-1.165	-1.640	1.602	

G = girls, B = Boys. Standard Deviations are presented in the parentheses.

*indicates significance at the level of $p<0.05$, ** indicates significance at the level of $p<0.01$ and *** indicates significance at the level of $p<0.001$.

The prevalence of age and sex wise nutritional status based on Cole et al., (2000 and 2007) cut offs of the studied children are presented in Table 3. The prevalence of overall thinness, overweight and obese for girls was 50.6%, 4.4% and 0.9%, respectively. The corresponding prevalence was 46.2%, 5.2% and 1.6% for boys overall thinness, overweight and obese, respectively. Overall, 44.1% of the studied girls were found to be normal category followed by thinness grade I with 30.2%, thinness grade II with 11.8%, thinness grade III with 8.6%, overweight with 4.4% and obese with 0.9%.In case of boys, 47.0% were observed to be normal category followed by thinness grade I with 25.7%, thinness grade II with 13.7%, thinness grade III with 6.8%, overweight with 5.2% and obese with 1.6%. The prevalence of overall thinness, normal, overweight and obese for age and sex combined were 48.5%, 45.4%, 4.85% and 1.2%, respectively. Results of χ^2 test revealed that there were no age group and sex wise significant differences in prevalence of nutritional status except in overweight category ($\chi^2 = 9.538$, df = 4 and $p < 0.05$). Age combined sex differences in different grades of nutritional status were also not statistically significant ($\chi^2 = 4.112$; df = 5 and $p > 0.05$).

Table 3. Prevalence of age and sex wise nutritional status among studied children according to Cole et al., (2000 and 2007) cut offs of BMI

Age (Years)	Sex (n)	Thinness Grade III	Thinness Grade II	Thinness Grade I	Overall Thinness (III+II+I)	Normal	Over weight	Obese
6	G (n = 60)	5(8.3)	5(8.3)	23(38.3)	33(54.9)	25(41.7)	1(1.7)	1(1.7)
	B (n = 51)	5(9.8)	7(13.7)	13(25.5)	25(49.0)	23(45.1)	2(3.9)	1(2.0)
7	G (n = 96)	10(10.4)	13(13.5)	26(27.1)	49(51.0)	40(41.7)	6(6.3)	1(1.0)
	B (n = 88)	6(6.8)	13(14.8)	19(21.6)	38(43.2)	4854.5)	2(2.3)	-
8	G (n = 116)	6(5.2)	15(12.9)	34(29.3)	55(47.4)	58(50.0)	2(1.7)	1(0.9)
	B (n = 97)	5(5.2)	8(8.2)	26(26.8)	39(40.2)	47(48.5)	10(10.3)	1(1.0)
9	G (n = 108)	11(10.1)	15(13.9)	30(27.8)	56(51.8)	45(41.7)	6(5.6)	1(0.9)
	B (n = 95)	4(4.2)	16(16.8)	24(25.3)	44(46.3)	43(45.3)	5(5.3)	3(3.1)
10	G (n = 51)	5(9.8)	3(6.0)	17(33.3)	25(49.1)	22(43.1)	4(7.8)	-
	B (n = 50)	6(12.0)	8(16.0)	16(32.0)	30(60.0)	18(36.0)	1(2.0)	1(2.0)
Total	G (n = 431)	37(8.6)	51(11.8)	130(30.2)	218(50.6)	190(44.1)	19(4.4)	4(0.9)
	B (n = 381)	26(6.8)	52(13.7)	98(25.7)	176(46.2)	179(47.0)	20(5.2)	6(1.6)
	$\chi 2$	2.607	4.759	1.162	2.665	2.082	9.538*	2.708
Overall	n = 812	63(7.8)	103(12.7)	228(28.1)	394(48.5)	369(45.4)	39(4.8)	10(1.2)

G = girls and B = boys. Percentages are presented in the parentheses.*Means significance at the level of p<0.05.

DISCUSSION

Child growth monitoring is universally used to assess nutrition, health and development of individual children, and to estimate the overall nutritional status and health of populations (WHO, 1995).The prevalence of undernutrition among children and adolescents remains an enduring public health concern in developing countries like India (Nandy et al., 2005). Hitherto, India still remains as the country facing with the largest burden of undernutrition while the rates of overnutrition are also gradually increasing (IFPRI, 2015).

Our investigation assessed the nutritional status based on BMI cut offs among rural children of Hooghly District, West Bengal, India. It was observed from present study that half of the studied girls (50.6%) were undernourished (or suffered from thinness). In our study, we found that the age and sex combined prevalence of overall thinness, overweight and obese were 48.5%, 4.8% and 1.2%, respectively. Underweight and thinness were observed as the most profound forms of malnutrition in populations of South-East Asia and Africa while in Latin America this problem is less (generally below 10%) prevalence of underweight or thinness (Best et al., 2010). It was observed that girls were thinner than boys (girls 50.6% vs. boys 46.2%). Similar findings was observed by numerous previous researchers from West Bengal state (Das and Bose, 2011a; Das and Bose, 2011b; Das et al., 2012a; Mandal and Bose, 2014; and Das et al., 2015), other states of India (Sikdar, 2012; Singh et al., 2015; Bartwal, 2017; and Chudasama et al., 2017), and also abroad (Caleyachetty et al., 2012; Rana et al., 2012; Mustaq et al., 2012; Wamba et al., 2013; Akinpelu et al., 2014; Schonbeck et al., 2014; O'Dea et al., 2014; Zhang et al., 2016; and Partap et al., 2017). However, Chakraborty and Bose (2009), Bisai et al., (2010), Mondal and Sen (2010), Mondal et al., (2011), Das et al., (2012b), Debnath et al., (2018) and Pal and Bose (communicated) from different districts of West Bengal; Singh and Mondal (2013), Longkumar (2013), Mondal et al.,(2015), Bharthi et al., (2017), and Das et al., (2017) from other different states of India; and Bovet et al., (2011) from Seychelles and Ejike et al., (2013) from Nigeria reported different findings that boys were more affected by thinness than girls. Comparison of the prevalence of thinness of present study with other studies (Chakraborty and Bose, 2009; Bisai et al., 2010; Mondal and Sen, 2010; Das and Bose, 2011a; Mondal et al., 2011; Das et al., 2011b; Das et al., 2012a; Das et al., 2012b; Mandal and Bose, 2014; Das et al., 2015; Das et al., 2017; Debnath et al., 2018 and Pal and Bose [communicated]) from West Bengal is presented in Table 4. Here, we considered only those studies for comparison who have utilized Cole et al., (2000 and 2007) cut-offs of BMI for evaluating the nutritional status. Previous regional studies (from West Bengal) have reported higher rates of overall thinness except findings of Das and Bose, (2011a) among Santal children and adolescents of Purulia districts. Table 5 shows the comparison of the prevalence of thinness with other studies (Sikdar, 2012; Bansal and Joshi, 2013; Singh and Mondal, 2013; Longkumar, 2013; Singh et al., 2014; Mondal et al., 2015; Singh et al., 2015; Das et al., 2016; Bharthi et al., 2017; Bartwal, 2017; Das et al., 2017 and Chudasama et al., 2017) from India. All studies from different states of India have found lower rates of overall thinness than the present study except Singh et al., (2015). A study conducted by Chudasama et al., (2017) among urban affluent school children from Rajkot city of Gujrat reported low (3.3%) prevalence of thinness when compared with regional and national studies. Comparison of the prevalence of thinness of present study with other studies (da Silva et al., 2008; Bovet et al., 2011; Ene-Obong et al., 2012; Caleyachetty et al., 2012; Rana et al., 2012; Mustaq et al., 2012; Ejike et al., 2013; Wamba et al., 2013; Akinpelu et al., 2014; Schonbeck et al., 2014; O'Dea et al., 2014; Zhang et al., 2016 and Partap et al., 2017) from the world is presented in table 6. All studies from other countries of the world observed lower rates of thinness than prevalence of the present study.

Table 4. Comparison of the prevalence of thinness of present study with other studies from West Bengal (Thinness evaluation method as per Cole et al., 2007 cut-offs)

Study children	Study area	Age group (years)	Total sample size (n)	Thinness prevalence (%)			Reference
				B	G	O	
Rural primary school children	Nandigram, Purba Medinipur District, West Bengal, India	5-10	T-596 B-315 G-281	62.9	61.6	-	Chakraborty and Bose, 2009
Kora-Mudi tribal children	Paschim Medinipur District, West Bengal, India	2-13	T-119 B-59 G-60	67.8	66.7	67.2	Bisai et al., 2010
Rural primary school children	Phansidewa Block of Darjeeling District, West Bengal, India	5-12	T-2111 B-1028 G-1083	71.11	67.77	-	Mondal and Sen, 2010
Santal tribal children and adolescents	Purulia District, West Bengal, India	7-18	T-421 B-214 G-204	38.2	44.6	41.3	Das and Bose, 2011a
Rural Bengalee Muslim school children	Chapra Block of Nadia District, West Bengal, India	6-16	T-642 B-308 G-334	58.77	54.79	56.7	Mondal et al., 2011
Hill Kharia tribal children	Purulia, West Bengal, India	4-18	T-136 B-71 G-65	52.2	53.8	52.9	Das and Bose, 2011b
Birhor tribal children	Bhupatipalli and Bareriya villages of Baghmundi Block, Purulia	7-12	T-30 B-15 G-15	66.6	86.7	-	Das et al., 2012a
Rural primary school	Kharagpur of Paschim Medinipur, West Bengal, India	6-12	T-500 B-250 G-250	77.6	76.4	77.0	Das et al., 2012b
Santal primary school children	Bali Gram Panchayet of Arambagh, Hooghly District, West Bengal, India	6-10	T-108 B-58 G-50	75.9	76.0	75.95	Mandal and Bose, 2014
Rural children and adolescents	Paschim Medinipur, West Bengal, India	6-16	T-360 B-180 G-180	67.2	71.6	-	Das et al., 2015
Bengalee children	Two districts of West Bengal, India	2-12	T-2310 B-1144 G-1166	62.2	62.6	62.4	Das et al., 2017
Rural school children	Phansidewa Block of Darjeeling District, West Bengal, India	5-12	T-1250 B-618 G-632	65.53	47.94	57.36	Debnath et al., 2018

Table 4. (Continued)

Study children	Study area	Age group (years)	Total sample size (n)	Thinness prevalence (%)			Reference
				B	G	O	
Rural primary school children	Jangipara Block of Hooghly District, West Bengal, India	6-10	T-303 B-144 G-159	74.3	71.1	72.6	Pal and Bose (communicated)
Rural primary school children	Jangipara Block of Hooghly District, West Bengal, India	6-10	T-812 B-381 G-431	46.2	50.6	48.5	Present study

T, B, G and O stand for total, boys, girls, and overall, respectively.

Table 5. Comparison of the prevalence of thinness of present study with other studies from India (Thinness evaluation method as per Cole et al., 2007 cut-offs)

Study children	Area	Age group (years)	Total sample size (n)	Thinness prevalence (%)			Reference
				B	G	O	
Mishing tribal children	Assam, India	6-10	T-511 B-256 G-255	17.57	19.21	-	Sikdar, 2012
Sunni Muslim school girls	Delhi, India	6-12	G-370	-	38.37	-	Bansal and Joshi, 2013
Sonowal Kachari tribal children & adolescents	Dibrugarh District, Assam, India	6-18	T-1343 B-670 G-673	28.08	23.92	25.99	Singh and Mondal, 2013
Ao Naga tribal children	Mokokchung town, Nagaland	8-15	T-571 B-289 G-282	34.26	25.89	30.12	Longkumar, 2013
Bhaina tribal girls	Pendra District, Chhattisgarh	6-12	T-28	-	57.1	-	Singh et al., 2014
Bodo tribal children	Udalguri District, Assam, India	5-11	T-1017 B-528 G-489	11.93	10.02	-	Mondal et al., 2015
Gond tribal children	Malnadih village of Karra Gram Panchayet, Bilaspur, Chattisgarh	6-12	T-91 B-47 G-44	51.1	52.3	51.7	Singh et al., 2015**
Bhaina tribal children	Pendra Block, Bilaspur District, Chattisgarh	7-12	T-26	-	53.8	-	Das et al., 2016

Table. 5 (Continued)

Study children	Area	Age group (years)	Total sample size (n)	Thinness prevalence (%)			Reference
				B	G	O	
Kolam tribal children & adolescents	Adilabad District, Telangana, India	6-18	T-827 B-413 G-414	62.9	40.3	-	Bharthi et al., 2017
Bhotia tribal children & adolescents	Chamoli and Uttarakashi Districts of Uttarakhand, India.	6-18	T-643 B-336 G-307	7.44	13.03		Bartwal, 2017
Urban school children	Faridabad district, Haryana	5-10	T-5643 B-3300 G-2343	30.0	29.5	-	Das et al., 2017
Urban affluent school children	Rajkot city, Gujrat	8-18	T-1496 B-1183 G-313	3.1	4.2	3.3	Chudasama et al., 2017
Rural primary school children	Jangipara Block, Hooghly District, West Bengal, India	6-10	T-812 B-381 G-431	46.2	50.6	48.5	Present study

T, B, G and O stand for total, boys, girls, and overall, respectively.

** Here we pooled the percentage prevalence (thinness grade I, grade II and grade III).

Table 6. Comparison of the prevalence of thinness of present study with other studies from World (Thinness evaluation method as per Cole et al., 2007 cut-offs)

Study children	Area	Age group (years)	Total sample size (n)	Thinness prevalence (%)			Reference
				B	G	O	
Public School children	Rio de Janeiro, Brazil	7-9	T-160 B-91 G-69	0.0	0.0	0.0	da Silva et al., 2008
School children	Seychelles	5-16*	T-33340 B-16672 G-16668	30.3	29.2	29.8**	Bovet et al., 2011
Urban children & adolescents	Four towns (Lagos, Port Harcourt, Nsukka, and Aba), Nigeria	5-18	T-1599 B-796 G-803	-	-	13.0	Ene-Obong et al., 2012
Primary school children	Mauritius	9-10	T-841 B-412 G-429	12.4	13.1	-	Caleyachetty et al., 2012

Table 6. (Continued)

Study children	Area	Age group (years)	Total sample size (n)	Thinness prevalence (%)			Reference
				B	G	O	
Garo tribal children	Sherpur District, Bangladesh	5-10	T-324 B-175 G-149	30.85	31.53	30.88	Rana et al., 2012
Primary school children	Lahore, Pakistan	5-12	T-1860 B-977 G-883	26.7	30.2	28.4	Mustaq et al., 2012**
Primary and secondary school children	Umuahia, capital city of Abia State, Nigeria	7-17	T-1911 B-931 G-980	17.3	15.5	-	Ejike et al., 2013
School children	Cameroon	8-15	T-2689 B-1285 G-1404	9.4	9.7	9.5	Wamba et al., 2013
School children	Lagos State, Nigeria	1-10	T-1903 B-940 G-963	39.7	46.0	42.9	Akinpelu et al., 2014**
Children and adolescents	Netherlands	2-18	T-6620 B-3125 G-3495	9.5	10.1	-	Schonbeck et al., 2014
Children and adolescents	Australia	6-18	T-12443 B-6630 G-5813	4.6	6.0	-	O'Dea et al., 2014
School children	Shandong, China	7-18	T-42348 B-21248 G-21100	9.8	15.1	-	Zhang et al., 2016
Children	Segamat district, Johor State, Malaysia	6-18	T-6414 B-3174 G-3240	12.7	16.1	13.1	Partap et al., 2017
Rural primary school children	Jangipara Block, Hooghly District, West Bengal, India	6-10	T-812 B-381 G-431	46.2	50.6	48.5	Present study

T, B, G and O stand for total, boys, girls, and overall, respectively. * Exact age group in years 5.5, 9.2, 12.5 and 15.7. ** Here we pooled the percentage prevalence (thinness grade I, grade II and grade III).

In the present study, boys were more affected by obesity than girls. The prevalence of overweight was 5.2% and 4.4% among boys and girls, respectively. Obesity prevalence among boys and girls was 1.6% and 0.9%, respectively. In India, several previous studies (Chatterjee, 2002; Sidhu et al., 2006; Marwaha et al., 2006; Bose et al., 2007; Sharma et al.,

2007; Kaur et al., 2008; Khadilkar et al., 2011; Mishra et al., 2011; Ghosh et al., 2011; Siddiqui and Bose, 2012; Singh and Devi, 2013; Longkumar, 2013; Sonya et al., 2014; Mondal et al., 2015; and Eshwar et al., 2017) had observed different magnitudes of overweight and obesity among children and adolescents. Similarly, numerous studies (Kapil et al., 2002; Ramachandran et al., 2002; Subramanyam et al., 2003; Mohan et al., 2004; Khadilkar and Khadilkar, 2004; Gupta et al., 2006; Kaneria et al., 2006; Iyer et al., 2006; Sood et al., 2007; Rao et al., 2007; Laxmaiah et al., 2007; Unnithan and Syamakumari, 2007; Goyal et al., 2010; Alok et al., 2012; Bisai et al., 2012; Mandal (Nandi) and Mandal, 2012 and Pawar et al., 2016) also confirmed the presence of overnutrition among adolescents of India.

Some of the limitations of our study were the small sample size from a limited study area. Moreover, it was cross-sectional in nature.

Conclusion

In conclusion, our study clearly indicated that half of the studied girls (50.6%) were undernourished and boys were affected to be overweight and obese. Our investigation stated that rural children were experienced very high prevalence of malnutrition. More studies should be conducted among children utilizing the same international cut-offs of BMI. Regular periodic surveillance of growth and nutritional status of children are required for early detection of malnutrition and growth faltering. Surveillance of present nutritional schemes and state specific appropriate and immediate new nutritional interventions are required to ameliorate the problem of malnutrition.

Acknowledgments

All participants and school authorities are gratefully acknowledged for their cooperation during data collection. The first author also expresses sincere gratitude to her parents for all their support during data collection. The University Grants Commission of India is also sincerely acknowledged for the financial assistance in the form of Senior Research Fellowship (Ref. No.: 590/ (NET/DEC.2013) to the first author.

AUTHOR'S CONTRIBUTION

SP and KB conceptualized and designed the study. SP collected and analysed the data. SP prepared the first draft and KB edited the draft.

CONFLICTS OF INTEREST

Authors hereby declare that there are no conflicts of interests.

REFERENCES

Akinpelu, A. O., O. O. Oyewole, A. C. Odole, and B. A. Tella. "Nutritional status of Nigerian children from urban community using different reference cut-offs." *African Journal of Biomedical Research* 17, no. 2 (2014): 61-67.

Alok, P., P. Malay, and V. Divyeshkumar. "Prevalence of overweight and obesity in adolescents of urban and rural area of Surat, Gujarat." *National Journal of Medical Research* 2, no. 3 (2012): 325-29.

Banik, S. D., and S. Chatterjee. "Nutritional status of school going children and adolescents aged 9-13 years at Haldia in West Bengal, India." *Paediatrica Indonesiana* 50, no. 3 (2010): 159-65.

Bansal, A., and P.C. Joshi. "Manifestation of malnutrition among Sunni Muslim Girls of Delhi (6-12 years)." *Journal of Human Sciences* 10, no. 1 (2013): 1128-1134.

Bartwal, S. M. "Nutritional health status of Bhotia tribal children of Uttarakhand, India." In: *Child Health in India*, edited by Bhaskar Das,

Moromi Talukdar and Anup Jyoti Bharali, 120-129. New Delhi: Omsons Publications, 2017.

Best, C., N. Neufingerl, L. van Geel, T. van den Briel, and S. Osendarp. "The nutritional status of school-aged children: why should we care?." *Food and Nutrition Bulletin* 31, no. 3 (2010): 400-417.

Bharthi, K., M. Ghritlahre, S. Das, and K. Bose. "Nutritional status among children and adolescents aged 6–18 years of Kolam tribe of Andhra Pradesh, India." *Anthropological Review* 80, no. 2 (2017): 153-163.

Bisai, S., R. Khongsdier, K. Bose, and D. Mahalanabis. "Double burden of malnutrition among urban Bengalee adolescent boys in Midnapore, West Bengal, India." *Nature Precedings [http://hdl. handle. net/10101/npre. 2012.7106. 1]*(2012).

Bisai, S., T. Ghosh, G. K. De, and K. Bose. "Very high prevalence of thinness among Kora Mudi tribal children of Paschim Medinipur District of West Bengal, India." *EJ Biol Sci* 3, no. 1 (2010): 43-9.

Black, R. E., C. G. Victora, S. P. Walker, Z. A. Bhutta, P. Christian, M. de Onis, M. Ezzati, S. Grantham-McGregor, J. Katz, R. Martorell, R. Uauy, and the Maternal and Child Nutrition Study Group. "Maternal and child undernutrition and overweight in low-income and middle-income countries." *The Lancet* 382, no. 9890 (2013): 427-4512013. http://dx.doi.org/10.1016/S0140-6736(13)60937-X.

Black, R. E., L. H. Allen, Z. A. Bhutta, L. E. Caulfield, M. de Onis, M. Ezzati, C. Mathers, J. Rivera, and the Maternal and Child Undernutrition Study Group. "Maternal and child undernutrition: global and regional exposures and health consequences." *The Lancet* 371, no. 9608 (2008): 243-260. doi: 10.1016/S0140-6736(07)61690-0.

Bose, K., S. Bisai, A. Mukhopadhyay, and M. Bhadra. "Overweight and obesity among affluent Bengalee schoolgirls of Lake Town, Kolkata, India." *Maternal and child Nutrition* 3, no. 2 (2007): 141-45.

Bovet, P., N. Kizirian, G. Madeleine, M. Blossner, and A. Chiolero. "Prevalence of thinness in children and adolescents in the Seychelles: comparison of two international growth references." *Nutrition Journal* 10, no. 1 (2011): 65. Doi: 10.1186/1475-2891-10-65.

Caleyachetty, R., A. R. Rudnicka, J. B. Echouffo-Tcheugui, K. R. Siegel, N. Richards, and P. H. Whincup. "Prevalence of overweight, obesity and thinness in 9-10 year old children in Mauritius." *Globalization and Health* 8, no. 1 (2012): 28. Doi: 10.1186/1744-8603-8-28.

Chakraborty, R., and K. Bose. "Very high prevalence of thinness using new international body mass index cut off points among 5-10 year old school children of Nandigram, west Bengal, India." *Journal of research in medical sciences: the official journal of Isfahan University of Medical Sciences* 14, no. 2 (2009): 129-133.

Chatterjee, P. "India sees parallel rise in mal-nutrition and obesity." *Lancet* 360, no. 9349 (2002): 1948.

Chudasama, R.K., T. K. M. Eshwar, D. Thakrar, and S. T. Eshwar. "Prevalence and comparison of obesity, overweight, and thinness by different growth standards among affluent school children (8–18 years) in Rajkot." *Journal of Mahatma Gandhi Institute of Medical Sciences* 22, no. 2 (2017): 99-104. doi:10.4103/jmgims.jmgims_31_16. 2017.

Cole, T. J., M. C. Bellizzi, K. M. Flegal, and W. H. Dietz. "Establishing a standard definition for child overweight and obesity worldwide: international survey." *British Medical Journal* 320, no. 7244 (2000): 1240.

Cole, T.J., K. M. Flegal, D. Nicholls, and A. A. Jackson. "Body mass index cut offs to define thinness in children and adolescents: international survey." *British Medical Journal* 335, no. 7612 (2007): 194. Doi:10.1136/bmj.39238.399444.55.

da Silva, H. G., V. L. Chiara, M. E. Barros, A. L. Rêgo, A. Ferreira, B. A. Pitasi, and T. Mattos. "Diagnosing the nutritional status of school children: a comparison between Brazilian and international criteria." *Jornal de Pediatria* 84, no.6 (2008): 550-555.

Das, M. K., V. Bhatia, and A. Sibal. "Prevalence of Overweight and Obesity among Urban School Children Aged 5 to 10 Years in North India." *Index Copernicus International* 6, no. 4 (2017): 210-215.

Das, S., and K. Bose. "Prevalence of thinness using new international cut-off points among Santal tribal children and adolescents of

PuruliaDistrict, West Bengal, India." *Sri Lanka Journal of Child Health* 40, no. 3 (2011a): 105-110.

Das, S., and K. Bose. "Thinness among Hill Kharia Children and Adolescents of Purulia Using Body Mass Index Cut-Off Points." *Research & Reviews: A Journal of Health Professions* 1, no. 2 (2011b.): 31-36.

Das, S., D. Addhya, and F. Chakrabarty. "Prevalence of thinness among 6-12 years rural children of Kharagpur." *Anthrocom Journal of Anthropology* 8, no. 1 (2012b): 5-10.

Das, S., H. S. Singh, B. Tiwari, and K. Bose. "Evaluation of Undernutrition using International Cut-offs among 2-12 years children of Midnapore and Purulia, West Bengal, India." In: *Child Health in India*, edited by Bhaskar Das, Moromi Talukdar and Anup Jyoti Bharali, 1-12. New Delhi: Omsons Publications, 2017.

Das, S., M. Ghritlahre, B. Tiwari, and K. Bose. "Assessment of nutritional status among 2 to 12 years children of two districts in West Bengal, India." *Journal of Life Sciences* 9, no. 2 (2017a): 118-125.

Das, S., M. Gritlahre, H. S. Singh, S. D. Banik, and K. Bose. "Selected Socio-demographic Correlates of Nutritional Status among Bhaina Tribal Female Children and Women of Pendra Block, Chhattisgarh." *South Asian Anthropologist* 16, no. 1 (2016): 19-26.

Das, S., M. Mahata, and K. Bose. "Age-trend in thinness among Birhor children and adolescents of Purulia: a primitive tribe of West Bengal, India." *Asian Journal of Biological and life Sciences* 1, no. 1 (2012a): 58-60.

Das, S., S. Panda, and K. Bose. "Ethnic-Specific Prevalence of Thinness among Bengalee Youths of Midnapore, West Bengal, India." *Research Journal of Pharmaceutical Biological and Chemical Sciences* 6, no. 1 (2015): 1374-1380.

Debnath, S., N. Mondal, and J. Sen. "Prevalence of thinness among rural children of West Bengal, India." *Human Biology Review* 7, no. 4 (2018): 362-385.

Ejike, C. E. C. C., J. N. Onyemairo, and I. A. Onukogu. "Coexistence of child and adolescent obesity and thinness in a city in Nigeria:

Comparison of results derived from different reference standards." *International Journal of Nutrition, Pharmacology, Neurological Diseases* 3, no. 3 (2013): 276-81. Doi: 10.4103/2231-0738.114856.

Ene-Obong, H., V. Ibeanu, N. Onuoha, and A. Ejekwu. "Prevalence of overweight, obesity, and thinness among urban school-aged children and adolescents in southern Nigeria." *Food and Nutrition Bulletin 33,* no. 4 (2012): 242-250.

Eshwar, T. K. M., R. K. Chudasama, S. T. Eshwar, and D. Thakrar. "Prevalence of obesity and overweight and their comparison by three growth standards among affluent school students aged 8–18 years in Rajkot." *Indian Journal of Public Health* 61, no. 1 (2017): 51-54. doi: 10.4103/0019-557X.200251.

Food and Agricultural Organization office of evaluation. "Evaluation of FAO's Role and Work in Nutrition." Final Report. PC 108/6. Rome. 2011.

Food and Agriculture Organization of the United Nations. "The State of Food and Agriculture: Food systems for better Nutrition." 2013. Available online at: http://www.fao.org/docrep/018/i3300e/i3300e.pdf, accessed 2nd May 2019.

Ghosh, A. "Rural–urban comparison in prevalence of overweight and obesity among children and adolescents of Asian Indian origin." *Asia Pacific Journal of Public Health* 23, no. 6 (2011): 928-935.

Goyal, R. K., V. N. Shah, B. D. Saboo, S. R. Phatak, N. N. Shah, M. C. Gohel, P. B. Raval, and S. S. Patel. "Prevalence of overweight and obesity in Indian adolescent school going children: its relationship with socioeconomic status and associated lifestyle factors." *The Journal of the Association of Physicians of India* 58, (2010): 151-158.

Gupta, R., P. Rastogi, and S. Arora. "Low obesity and high undernutrition prevalence in lower socioeconomic status school girls: a double jeopardy." *Human Ecology* 14, no. 14 (2006): 65-70.

Hakim, M. A., and A. Rahman. Health and nutritional condition of street children of Dhaka city: an empirical study in Bangladesh. *Science Journal of Public Health 4, no.* 1, (2016), 6-9.

Hasan, N., M. Ashraf and A. Rahman. Effects of information communication technology (ICT) in the childhood developments and lives of disabilities: A multivariate analysis. *Science Journal of Public Health 4, no.* 1, (2016), 28-37. https://doi.org/10.11648/j.sjph.s.2016040101.15.

International Food Policy Research Institute. "Global Nutrition Report 2015: Actions and Accountability to Advance Nutrition and Sustainable Development." Washington, DC. Available online at http://ebrary.ifpri.org/utils/getfile/collection/p15738coll2/id/129443/filename/129654.pdf, accessed 2nd May 2019.

International Institute of Population Sciences (IIPS). "*National Family Health Survey (NFHS-4).*" 2015-2016. Available online at http://rchiips.org/nfhs/pdf/NFHS4/WB_FACTSheet.Pdf,Accessed on 17th December 2018.

Iyer, U. M., S. Venugopal, and H. I. Gandhi. "*Obesity in school children. Magnitude and risk factor analysis.*" ICMR funded project report, Department of Foods and Nutrition. WHO Collaborating Centre for Diet Related Non-Communicable Diseases and Anemia Control. Baroda: MS University of Baroda, India, (2006).

Kaneria, Y., P. Singh, and D. C. Sharma. "Prevalence of overweight and obesity in relation to socio-economic conditions in two different groups of school-age children of Udaipur city (Rajasthan)." *Journal, Indian Academy of Clinical Medicine* 7, no. 2 (2006): 133-35.

Kapil, U., P. Singh, P. Pathak, S. N. Dwivedi, and S. Bhasin. "Prevalence of obesity in affluent adolescent school children in Delhi." *Indian Pediatrics* 39, no. 5 (2002): 449-52.

Kaur, S., H. P. S. Sachdev, S. N. Dwivedi, R. Lakshmy, and U. Kapil. "Prevalence of overweight and obesity amongst school children in Delhi, India." *Asia Pacific Journal of Clinical Nutrition* 17, no. 4 (2008): 592-596.

Khadilkar, V. V., A. V. Khadilkar, T. J. Cole, S. A. Chiplonkar, and D. Pandit. "Overweight and obesity prevalence and body mass index trends in Indian children." *International Journal of Pediatric Obesity* 6, no. sup3 (2011): e216-224.

Khadilkar, V. V., and A. V. Khadilkar. "Prevalence of obesity in affluent school boys in Pune." *Indian Pediatrics* 41, no. 8 (2004): 857-58.

Laxmaiah, A., B. Nagalla, K. Vijayaraghavan, and M. Nair. "Factors affecting prevalence of overweight among 12-to 17-year-old urban adolescents in Hyderabad, India." *Obesity* 15, no. 6 (2007): 1384-1390.

Lohman, T. G., A. F. Roche, and R. Martorell. *Anthropometric standardization reference manual.* Chicago: Human kinetics books, 1988.

Longkumar, T. "Physical growth and nutritional status among Ao Naga children of Nagaland, Northeast India." *Journal of Anthropology* 2013 (2013). http://dx.doi.org/10.1155/2013/291239.

Mandal (Nandi), A., and G. C. Mandal. "Prevalence of overweight and obesity among the urban adolescent English Medium School girls of Kolkata, India." *Italian Journal of Public Health* 9, no. 3 (2012): e7535-1 – 6.

Mandal, G. C., K. Bose, and S. Bisai. "Thinness among Rural Children in Bengal." *Indian Journal of Pediatrics* 76, no. 8 (2009): 817-819.

Mandal, G.C., and K. Bose. "Thinness among primary school children of the migrated Santals of Arambag, West Bengal, India." *International Journal of Food Safety, Nutrition and Public Health 5, no.* 1 (2014): 46-53.

Marwaha, R. K., N. Tandon, Y. Singh, R. Aggarwal, K. Grewal, and K. Mani. "A study of growth parameters and prevalence of overweight and obesity in school children from Delhi." *Indian Pediatrics* 43, no. 11 (2006): 943-52.

Megabiaw, B. and Rahman, A. Prevalence and determinants of chronic malnutrition among under-5 children in Ethiopia. *International Journal of Child Health and Nutrition 3, no.* 2, (2013), 230-236. https://doi.org/10.6000/1929-4247.2013.02.03.5.

Mengistu, K., K. Alemu, and B. Destaw. "Malnutrition and associated factors among children aged 6-59 months at Hidabu Abote district, North Shewa, Oromia regional state." *Journal Nutrition Disorder Therapy* (2013): 001.

Misra, A., P. Shah, K. Goel, D. K. Hazra, R. Gupta, Payal Seth, PoojaTallikotiet al., "The high burden of obesity and abdominal obesity in urban Indian schoolchildren: a multicentric study of 38,296 children." *Annals of Nutrition and Metabolism* 58, no. 3 (2011): 203-211.

Mohan, B., N. Kumar, N. Aslam, A. Rangbulla, S. Kumbkarni, N. K. Sood, and G. S. Wander. "Prevalence of sustained hypertension and obesity in urban and rural school going children in Ludhiana." *Indian Heart Journal* 56, no. 4 (2004): 310-314.

Mondal, N., and J. Sen. "Prevalence of undernutrition among children (5-12 years) belonging to three communities residing in a similar habitat in North Bengal, India." *Annals of Human Biology* 37, no. 2 (2010): 198-216.

Mondal, N., and J. Sen. "Thinness is a major underlying problem among Indian children." *Journal of Tropical Pediatrics 56, no.* 6 (2010): 456-58.

Mondal, N., B. Basumatary, J. Kropi, and K. Bose. "Prevalence of double burden of malnutrition among urban school going Bodo children aged 5-11 years of Assam, Northeast India." *Epidemiology, Biostatistics and Public Health* 12, no. 4 (2015): e114971-10.

Mondal, P. R., S. Biswas, and K. Bose. "Prevalence of thinness among rural Bengalee Muslim school children from eastern India." In: *Undernutrition Effects, causes, and management*. Edited by Jason E. Lee, 99-110. New York: Nova science publishers, Inc. 2011.

Mushtaq, M.U., S. Gull, K. Mushtaq, H. M. Abdullah, U. Khurshid, U. Shahid, M. A. Shad, and J. Akram. "Height, weight and BMI percentiles and nutritional status relative to the international growth references among Pakistani school-aged children." *BMC Pediatrics 12, no.* 1 (2012): 31.

Naing, L., T. Winn, and B. N. Rusli. "Practical issues in calculating the sample size for preventive studies." *Archives of orofacial Sciences* 1, (2006): 9-14.

Nandy, S., M. Irving, D. Gordon, S. V. Subramanian, and G. D. Smith. "Poverty, child undernutrition and morbidity: new evidence from

India." *Bulletin of the World Health Organization* 83, no. 3 (2005): 210-216.

O'Dea, J. A., and M. J. Dibley. "Prevalence of obesity, overweight and thinness in Australian children and adolescents by socioeconomic status and ethnic/cultural group in 2006 and 2012." *International Journal of Public Health* 59, no. 5 (2014): 819–828. Doi: https://doi.org/10.1007/s00038-014-0605-3.

Pal, S., and K. Bose. "Thinness among rural primary school children of Hooghly District, West Bengal, India." *North Bengal Anthropologist (annually)*, communicated.

Park, K. "*Park's textbook of preventive and social medicine*," 18th ed. Jabalpur: Banarasidas Bhanot Publishers, 2005.

Partap, U., E. H. Young, P. Allotey, M. S. Sandhu, D. D. Reidpath. "The Use of Different International References to Assess Child Anthropometric Status in a Malaysian Population." *The Journal of Pediatrics* 190, (2017): 63-68. https://doi.org10.1016/j.jpeds.2017.07.049.

Pawar, S. V., A. S. Choksey, S. S. Jain, R. G. Surude, and P. M. Rathi. "Prevalence of overweight and obesity in 4 schools of south Mumbai." *Journal of Clinical and Diagnostic Research* 10, no. 3 (2016): OC01-OC02. DOI: 10.7860/JCDR/2016/17624.7383.

Rahman, A. and C. S. Biswas. Nutritional status of under-5 children in Bangladesh. *South Asian Journal of Population and Health 2, no.* 1, (2009), 1-11.

Rahman, A. and S. Chowdhury. Determinants of chronic malnutrition among preschool children in Bangladesh. *Journal of Biosocial Science 39, no.* 2, (2007), 161-173. https://doi.org/10.1017/S0021932006001295.

Rahman, A. and M. A. Hakim. Malnutrition prevalence and health practices of homeless children: a cross-sectional study in Bangladesh. *Science Journal of Public Health 4, no.* 1, (2016a), 10-15.

Rahman, A. and A. Harding. Social and health costs of tobacco smoking in Australia: level, trend and determinants. *International Journal of Statistics and Systems 6, no.* 4, (2011), 399-411.

Rahman, A. and A. Harding. Prevalence of overweight and obesity epidemic in Australia: some causes and consequences. *JP Journal of Biostatistics 10, no.* 1, (2013), 31-48.

Rahman, A. and M. S. Rahman. Rural-urban differentials of childhood malnutrition in Bangladesh. *International Journal of Child Health and Nutrition* (2019), 35-42. https://doi.org/10.6000/1929-4247.2019.08.01.5.

Rahman, A. and M. Sapkota. Knowledge on vitamin A rich foods among mothers of preschool children in Nepal: Impacts on public health and policy concerns. *Science Journal of Public Health 2, no.* 4, (2014), 316-322. https://doi.org/10.11648/j.sjph.20140204.22.

Rahman, A. Significant risk factors for childhood malnutrition: Evidence from an Asian developing country. *Science Journal of Public Health 4, no.* 1, (2016), 16-27.

Rahman, A. Estimating small area health-related characteristics of populations: A methodological review. *Geospatial Health 12, no.* 1, (2017), 3-14. [495]. https://doi.org/10.4081/gh.2017.495.

Rahman, A. Geospatial, socioeconomic, demographic and health determinants of childhood mortality in Bangladesh. *Demography India: population - society - economy - environment - interactions 48, no.* 2, (2019), 74-85.

Rahman, A., and M. A. Hakim. Measuring modified mass energy equivalence in nutritional epidemiology: A proposal to adapt the biophysical modelling approach. *International Journal of Statistics in Medical Research 5, no.* 3, (2016b), 219-223.

Rahman, A., and M. A. Hakim. An epidemiological study on hygiene practice and malnutrition prevalence of beggars children in Bangladesh. *International Journal of Nutrition and Dietetics 4, no.* 1, (2016c), 29-46. https://doi.org/10.17654/ND004010029.

Rahman, A., S. Chowdhury, and D. Hossain. Acute malnutrition in Bangladeshi children levels and determinants. *Asia-Pacific Journal of Public Health 21, no.* 3, (2009), 294-302. https://doi.org/10.1177/10105 39509335399.

Rahman, A., S. Chowdury, A. Karim, and S. Ahmed. Factors associated with nutritional status of children in Bangladesh: A multivariate analysis. *Demography India: population - society - economy - environment - interactions 37, no.* 1, (2008), 95-109.

Rahman, A., M. A. Hakim, M. A. Hanif, M. R. Islam, and M. Kamruzzaman. Dietary practices, health status and hygiene observance of slum kids: A pilot study in an Asian developing country. *JP Journal of Biostatistics 13, no.* 2, (2016), 195-208. https://doi.org/10.17654/BO013020195.

Rahman, A., M. S. Rahman, and M. A. Rahman. Determinants of infant mortality in Bangladesh: A nationally surveyed data analysis. *International Journal of Child Health and Nutrition 8, no.* 3, (2019), 93-102. https://doi.org/10.6000/1929-4247.2019.08.03.3.

Ramachandran, A., C. Snehalatha, R. Vinitha, M. Thayyil, C. K. S. Kumar, L. Sheeba, S. Joseph, and V. Vijay. "Prevalence of overweight in urban Indian adolescent school children." *Diabetes Research and Clinical Practice* 57, (2002): 185–90.

Rana, M. M., A. Ferdoushi, S. Tamanna, F. Sabrin, and N. N. Afroz. "Assessment of nutritional status of 5-10 years Garo children in Sherpur District, Bangladesh." *International Journal of Biosciences 2, no.* 11 (2012): 66-73.

Rao, S., A. Kanade, and R. Kelkar. "Blood pressure among overweight adolescents from urban school children in Pune, India." *European Journal of Clinical Nutrition* 61, no. 5 (2007): 633-41.

Schönbeck, Y., P. van Dommelen, R. A. HiraSing, and S. van Buuren. "Thinness in the era of obesity: trends in children and adolescents in The Netherlands since 1980." *European Journal of Public Health* 25, no. 2 (2014): 268-73. Doi:10.1093/eurpub/cku.130.

Sharma, A., K. Sharma, and K. P. Mathur. "Growth pattern and prevalence of obesity in affluent school children of Delhi." *Public Health Nutrition* 10, no. 5 (2007): 485-491.

Siddiqui, N. I., and S. Bose. "Prevalence and trends of obesity in Indian school children of different socioeconomic class." *Indian Journal of Basic and Applied Medical Research* 5, (2012): 393-398.

Sidhu, S., N. Kaur, and R. Kaur. "Overweight and obesity in affluent school children of Punjab."*Annals of Human Biology* 33, no. 2 (2006): 255-259.http://doi.org/10.1080/0301440600578631.

Sikdar, M. "Prevalence of malnutrition among the Mising children of Northeast India: A comparison between four different sets of criteria." *North American Journal of Medical Sciences* 4, no. 7 (2012): 305-9. DOI: 10.4103/1947-2714.98589.

Singh, H. S., P. K. Das, S. Das, S. D. Banik, and K. Bose. "Sociodemographic profile and nutritional status of Gondtribals from Malanadih village, Chattisgarh." *American Journal of Advances in Medical Sciences* 3, no. 1 (2015): 22-29.

Singh, H.S., M. Ghritlahre, and S. Das. "Nutritional status among females of bhaina tribe of Bilaspur, Chhattisgarh, India: An Anthropological Insight." *Journal of Anthropology* 2014, (2014). http://dx.doi.org/10.1155/2014/897893.

Singh, J., and N. Mondal. "Assessment of nutritional status: A case of tribal children in Assam, Northeast India." *Journal of Nepal Paediatric Society* 33, no. 1 (2013): 1-7.

Singh, M. S., and R. K. N. Devi. "Nutritional status among the urban Meitei children and adolescents of Manipur, Northeast India." *Journal of Anthropology* 2013, (2013). http://dx.doi.org/10.1155/2013/983845.

Sonya, J., R. Harish, P. Miranda, R. Unnikrishnan, R. M. Anjana, and V. Mohan. "Prevalence of overweight and obesity among school children and adolescents in chennai." *Indian Pediatrics* 51, no. 7 (2014): 544-49.

Sood, A., P. Sundararaj, S. Sharma, A. V. Kurpad, and S. Muthayya. "BMI and body fat percent: affluent adolescent girls in Bangalore City." *Indian Paediatrics* 44, no. 8 (2007): 587-91.

Subramanyam, V., and M. Rafi. "Prevalence of overweight and obesity in affluent adolescent girls in Chennai in 1981 and 1998." *Indian Pediatrics* 40, no. 4 (2003): 332-336.

Sulthan, M. S. "Prevalence of stunting and thinness among school-age children of working and non-working mothers in rural areas of Aligarh

District." *Indian Journal of Basic and Applied Medical Research* 3, no. 3 (2014): 51-57.

Touitou, Y., F. Portaluppi, M. H. Smolensky, and L. Rensing. "Ethical principles and standards for the conduct of human and animal biological rhythm research." *Chronobiology International* 21, no. 1 (2004): 161-170.

Ulijaszek, S. J., and D. A. Kerr. "Anthropometric measurement error and the assessment of nutritional status." *British Journal of Nutrition* 82, no. 3 (1999): 165-77.

Unnithan, A., and S. Syamakumari. "Prevalence of overweight, obesity and underweight among school going children in rural and urban areas of Thiruvananthapuram Educational District, Kerala State (India)." *The Internet Journal of Nutrition and Wellness* 6, no. 2 (2008): 1-6.

Wamba, P. C. F., J. E. Oben, and K. Cianflone. "Prevalence of Overweight, Obesity, and Thinness in Cameroon Urban Children and Adolescents." *Journal of Obesity* 2013, (2013). http://dx.doi.org/10.1155/2013/737592.

World Health Organization. "Physical status: The use of and interpretation of anthropometry, Report of a WHO Expert Committee." *Technical Report Series No. 854*. Geneva: World Health Organization, (1995).

Zhang, Y., Z, Wang, M. Wang, and L. Xie. "Prevalence of thinness among children and adolescents in Shandong, China." *European Journal of Nutrition* 55, no. 2 (2016): 809-813. Doi: 10.1007/s00394-015-0902-5.

In: Malnutrition
Editor: Azizur Rahman
ISBN: 978-1-53617-597-4

Chapter 3

ASSOCIATED RISK FACTORS FOR ACUTE MALNUTRITION AMONG RURAL BANGLADESHI CHILDREN: A CROSS-SECTIONAL ANALYSIS

***Md. Ashfikur Rahman*[1,2*]*, Md. Sazedur Rahman*[3,4†]*, and Azizur Rahman*[5,‡]**

[1]College of Economics and Management,
Northwest A&F University, Shaanxi, China
[2]Development Studies Discipline, Khulna University,
Khulna, Bangladesh
[3]School of Public Health, Shandong University, Shandong, China
[4]Statistics Discipline, Khulna University, Khulna, Bangladesh
[5]School of Computing and Mathematics, Charles Sturt University,
Wagga Wagga, Australia

* Corresponding Author's Email: ashfikurr@gmail.com.
† Corresponding Author's Email: sazedur.stat@gmail.com.
‡ Corresponding Author's Email: azrahman@csu.edu.au.

ABSTRACT

Background: Childhood malnutrition is considered as a serious public health problem in Bangladesh. Low weight-for-height (wasting) is a significant indicator for acute malnutrition, and rural children in Bangladesh are more vulnerable to be acutely malnourished compared to their urban counterparts. This study aims to observe prevalence and the key determinants of acute malnutrition in rural children in Bangladesh.

Methods: To assess the prevalence and determinants of acute malnutrition in rural children aged under five years old in Bangladesh, this study used nationally representative data from the 2014 Bangladesh Demographic Health and Survey (BDHS. Chi-square test was performed to investigate the association between outcome variables and selected covariates. Multinomial logistic regression was used to identify significant factors associated with acute malnutrition.

Results: All the selected factors in this study were significant at p-value < 0.10 in Chi-square test. The overall estimated prevalence rate of acute malnutrition in rural Bangladeshi children was 16.7%; among them 12.2% were moderately wasted ($-3.0 \leq$ Z-score < -2.0) and 4.5% severely wasted (Z-score < -3.0). In the multinomial regression, being male children, smaller than average size at birth, low maternal BMI (≤ 18.50 kg/m^2), short maternal height (<145cm) and poor household were found to be significant determinants for acute malnutrition among children under five years old in rural Bangladesh.

Conclusion: Findings of this study clearly indicate that the prevalence of wasting among rural Bangladeshi children is quite high despite the country's economic development. Understanding of those factors might enable to design and targeting any preventive-intervention programs or policies towards stopping and improving the child acute malnutrition.

Keywords: acute malnutrition, wasting, undernutrition, under-5 years, Bangladesh

BACKGROUND

The government of Bangladesh deliberately integrates the health sector in the poverty reduction strategy or plans [1]. In the 47 years since independence in 1971, the entire health system has gone through a series of reformations [2] and Bangladesh has achieved admirable success in Millennium Development Goals (MDGs), particularly in declining child and maternal mortality [3-4]. However, still, there exist different problems related to public health issues. Childhood malnutrition is a common disease burden particularly for children under five years old around the world, and low-middle income countries like Bangladesh are of at great risk of it [5–7]. Because poor nutritional capacity has the obvious payoff of reducing child survivability even it may impede the way of physical and mental development of the children. These health conditions thus lead to a greater risk of transmissible diseases or critical infections which ultimately end in a higher economic burden of a society [8].

Around 50% of deaths among children under five (U5) years old are due to different forms of malnutrition [5–10]. Previous literature shows that malnutrition is positively correlated with poor physical and mental growth [5, 11], poor academic performance [5, 12-13], chronic diseases and low productivity in adulthood [13-14]. Although, over the last few decades Bangladesh has developed its economic sectors at a significant rate and it has not adequately influenced in improvements of child nutrition [15–17]. Still large number of children die each year in Bangladesh due to lack of adequate nutrition [18]. So, ensuring proper nutrition for all children is important because it affects the entire population.

In order to examine the general status of child health three anthropometric measurements such as height-for-age (stunting), weight-for-height (wasting) and weight-for-age (underweight) are widely recognized. Weight-for-height designates current nutritional status, and a child who is more than two standard deviations below (-2 SD) the reference median for weight-for-height is considered to be too thin for her or his height or wasting. Wasting is a significant indicator for acute malnutrition. Compared with other form of malnutrition, wasting is a stronger predictor for mortality in the children aged under five years old [5, 19]. For example, children with severe acute malnutrition (SAM) (which is defined as the weight-for-height measurement of 70% or less below the three standard deviation (-3 SD) of the reference median for weight-for-height [20]) are almost 9-folds higher at risk of dying than children without SAM [21]. The prevalence of wasting was about 8% in the children of under five years old throughout the world in 2011, although the rate was nearly double (about 15%) in south-central Asia [22]. The prevalence of wasting has remained constant at about 15% in Bangladesh since 2011 [7]. Vast literature supports that a wide range of variables can influence a child to be wasted. Previous studies in Bangladesh have revealed that gender [23-24], age [17, 25-26], birth weight [25, 27-28], place of residence [24, 29], measles vaccination [25], recent fever [24-25], maternal education [24], paternal education [30], maternal body mass index [16-17, 25, 27, 29], maternal age [24, 29] and household's wealth status [24] are significantly associated with acute malnutrition among children under five years old.

Place of residence is a significant determinant of childhood malnutrition [31-32]. Rural children in Bangladesh are more vulnerable to be acutely malnourished compared to their urban counterparts [4, 7, 16]. For instance, in 2014, the prevalence of wasting was about 13% among children in urban area whereas in rural area children the prevalence was about 17% [7]. But researchers have not directed their attention toward acute malnutrition research among children aged under five years old in rural Bangladesh using nationally representative data. This study aims to observe prevalence and the key determinants of acute malnutrition in rural children in Bangladesh using the 2014BDHS dataset, and to help policymakers to reduce the overall burden of acute malnutrition in rural children.

The outline of this paper is as follows. The information about the research materials and methods including data sources, outcome variables, predictor variables, and statistical analysis have discussed in methods section. Then overall analyses are presented and described in the results section. Discussion section sets out a detailed discussion about the significant findings. The conclusion section highlights some final remarks with policy implications.

METHODS

Data Sources

The data for this study was extracted from the 2014 Bangladesh Demographic and Health Survey (2014 BDHS), which was a cross-sectional survey conducted from June 28, 2014, to November 9, 2014, across the country [33]. The 2014 BDHS was the seventh national-level demographic and health survey through a collaborative effort of the National Institute of Population Research and Training (NIPORT), ICF International, USA, and Mitra & Associates as a part of the worldwide DHS program to provide nationally representative, updated and reliable estimates of health indicators.

The sampling frame was obtained from the list of enumeration areas (EAs) of the 2011 Population and Housing Census. In 2014, Bangladesh was divided into seven administrative divisions and each of which was divided into a number of districts and for the purposes of local government, each district was divided into a number of Upazila. Each urban area in an Upazila was divided into wards and mohallas whereas a rural area in an Upazila was divided into Union Parishad (UPs) and Mouzas.

The 2014 BDHS used two-stage stratified sampling design in both rural and urban areas. In the first stage, 600 EAs were selected with probability proportional to the EA size, with 207 EAs in urban areas and 393 in rural areas. In the second stage of sampling, a systematic sample of thirty households on average was selected per EA in urban and rural areas. From the expected 18000 households, 17863 ever-married women age 15-49 were interviewed with a response rate of 98 percent. A total of 7886 children's information were available in the 2014 BDHS where 5398(68.45%) children were from rural areas. Among the 5398 subjects, 517 were excluded due to a huge missing case and finally 4881 children included in this study for further data analysis.

Outcome Variable

The indicator weight-for-height was the main outcome variable to measuring acute malnutrition in this study. On the basis of Z-score of weight-for-height (WHZ) a child was categorized into: nourished (Z-score ≥ −2.0), moderately wasted (-3.0 ≤ Z-score < -2.0), and severely wasted (Z-score < -3.0). The Z-scores were calculated using the WHO AnthroPlus Software (version 3.2.2, 2011) from the age, height and weight of the children.

Independent Variables

The following independent variables were considered in this study: division; sex of child; child age (0-11 months, 12-21 months, 22-34 months, 35-59 months); size at birth (<average, ≥average), vitamin A in first 6 months, measles vaccination in first 9 months, fever in 2 weeks, diarrhea in 2 weeks, maternal age at first birth (<20 years, ≥20 years), maternal BMI (≤ 18.50 kg/m^2, >18.50 kg/m2), maternal height (<145 cm, ≥145 cm), maternal and paternal education (no education, primary, secondary, and higher), maternal occupation (household, agriculture sector, non-agriculture sector, service sector); paternal occupation (agriculture sector, non-agriculture sector, business, and service sector); wealth index (poor, middle, rich); mother exposure to TV, toilet facilities (no facilities, hanging toilet, pit toilet, flush toilet); number of children aged under five years old children; and birth order.

Statistical analysis: Descriptive statistics was applied to report the background characteristics of the children according to the weight-for-height conditions. The individual association test also performed using Pearson's chi-square test. Then with the significant factors at $p \leq 0.05$ from the bivariate level, we used multinomial logistic regression models to estimate the odds ratio (OR) and 95% confidence intervals (CI) for any wasting conditions. Statistical Package for Social Science (SPSS Inc. Windows Version-23) was used for the analysis.

RESULTS

A total of 4881 rural children's information assessed in the study. The overall estimated prevalence rate of acute malnutrition in rural Bangladeshi children was 16.7%; among them 12.2% and 4.5% were moderately and severely wasted, respectively. Table 1 shows the individual background characteristics of children and the prevalence of wasting. About 51% children were female and about 12% of the children had a birth size that was smaller than average. Nearly 20% of the children were less than 1 year old, and the mean age of the study sample was approximately 29 months (SD = 17.11). More than 37% of the children had suffered from recent fever and around 5% had suffered from an episode of diarrhea. Also, nearly three-fourths (73%) of the children had been given measles vaccinations within their first 9 months of age. Besides, a quarter of the mothers had a low BMI ($\leq$18.50 kg/m^2), and almost 14% of mothers had height less than 145 cm. Only 28% of the children's mothers had been exposed to television. More than half (52%) of the families were poor and 3.32% of the household had no toilet facilities. Nearly 18% of the children lived in the Chittagong division, whereas about 17% and 15% resided in the Sylhet and Dhaka divisions, respectively.

Bivariate analyses (Table1) reveal that the prevalence of the moderate (12.7% vs. 11.6%) wasting was higher in the male children than the female. A similar result was also observed for the severe wasting (i.e., (5.4% for male vs. 3.5% for female). Moreover, the percentages of moderate and severe wasting were the highest among children aged less than 1 year (13.1% and 7.2%). Additionally, the percentage of children with moderate and severe wasting increases with decreasing levels of child's birth size, maternal BMI, maternal height and mother's exposure to television. For example, children whose birth size was less than average were 5.3% more moderately as well as 3.3% more severely wasted compared with their high-birth-size counterparts. Children who had not been given measles vaccinations had a higher percentage of for being severely wasted (6.8%) than their counterparts (3.6%). The prevalence rate of both moderate and severe wasting was the lowest (11.5% and 4.1%)

among children who had not suffered from recent fever. Similarly, the prevalence of both moderate and severe wasting was the lowest (12.0% and 4.4%) among children who were free from recent diarrhea. Furthermore, the prevalence of the both moderate and severe wasting was the highest among children from poor indexed household (13.6% and 5.5%). Similarly, children from the household without toilet facility had the highest percentage of moderately and severely wasted (19.1% and 6.2%). Finally, the prevalence of children with moderate wasting was the highest in the Rajshahi division (14.6%) and children with severe wasting was the highest in the Barisal division (6.1%).

The results of the multiple multinomial regression analysis are presented in Table 2. In this study, size at birth, maternal BMI and maternal height were significantly associated with moderate wasting; whereas sex of child, size at birth, maternal BMI, household wealth index and place of division were significantly associated with severe wasting.

The odds ratios show that the likelihood of the child being wasted increased with decreasing birth size, maternal BMI and maternal height. For example, children who had a smaller birth size than average were 1.61 and 1.71 times more likely to be moderately and severely wasted compared with children who had a larger than average birth size; the children of mothers with BMI $\leq$ 18.50 kg/m^2 had 1.71 times and 1.41 times higher odds for moderate and severe wasting than the children whose mothers had a BMI > 18.50 kg/m^2; and the children whose mothers had less than 145 cm height ran 1.25 times higher risk of becoming moderately wasted than the children whose mothers height was more than 145 cm. Male children were comparably possessed at a high risk of being severely wasted than their counterparts [OR = 1.62, 95% CI = 1.22-2.15), p = 0.001]. Besides, children from the poor household were 1.7-folds more likely to be severely wasted than the children from the rich household. Compared with the children of Dhaka division, the odds of severe and moderate wasting were significantly higher among the children of Barisal division (i.e., moderate [OR = 1.45, 95% CI = 1.03-2.02, p = 0.030], severe [OR = 2.30, 95% CI = 1.30-4.06, p = 0.004]) as well as children of Rajshahi division (i.e., moderate [OR = 1.45, 95% CI = 1.06-2.02, p = 0.026], severe wasting [OR

= 1.83, 95% CI = 1.02-3.31, *p* = 0.043]). Also, the children of Chittagong and Khulna division had 2.03 times and 1.96 times higher risk for severe wasting than the children of Dhaka division.

Table 1. Background characteristics of moderate and severe wasting children in rural Bangladesh (n = 4881)[1]

Characteristics	Overall[a] N (%)	Wasting		Nourished, N (%)	Chi-square value [df]
		Moderate, N (%)	Severe, N (%)		
Sex of child					12.72 [2]***
Male	2501(51.24)	317(12.7)	136(5.4)	2048(81.9)	
Female	2380(48.76)	277(11.6)	83(3.5)	2020(84.9)	
Child age (months)					29.09 [6]***
0-11	951(19.48)	125(13.1)	68(7.2)	758(79.7)	
12-21	874(17.91)	111(12.7)	47(5.4)	716(81.9)	
22-34	1042(21.35)	120(11.5)	39(3.7)	883(84.7)	
35-59	2014(41.26)	238(11.8)	65(3.2)	1711(85.0)	
Size at birth					28.78 [2]***
< Average	582 (11.9)	98 (16.8)	43(7.4)	441(75.8)	
≥ Average	4299(88.1)	496(11.5)	176(4.1)	3627(84.4)	
Measles vaccination in first 9 months					22.32 [2]***
No	1309(26.82)	155(11.8)	89(6.8)	1065(81.4)	
Yes	3572(73.18)	439(12.3)	130(3.6)	3003(84.1)	
Fever in 2 weeks					6.75 [2]**
No	3047(62.43)	349(11.5)	126(4.1)	2572(84.4)	
Yes	1834(37.57)	245(13.4)	93(5.1)	1496(81.6)	
Diarrhea in 2 weeks					7.69 [2]**
No	4643(95.12)	555(12.0)	203(4.4)	3026(65.17)	
Yes	238(4.88)	39(16.4)	16(6.7)	183(76.9)	
Maternal BMI (kg/m^2)					25.98 [2]***
≤ 18.50	1240(25.4)	190(15.3)	74(6.0)	976(78.7)	
>18.50	3641(74.6)	404(11.1)	145(4.0)	3092(84.9)	
Maternal height (cm)					5.94 [2]*
<145	672(13.8)	100(14.9)	33(4.9)	539(80.2)	
≥145	4209(86.2)	494(11.7)	186(4.4)	3529(83.8)	
Mother's exposure to television					15.03 [2]**
No	3496(71.62)	449(12.8)	176(5.0)	2871(82.1)	
Yes	1385(28.38)	145(10.5)	43(3.1)	1197(86.4)	
Wealth index					27.33 [4]***
Poor	2530(51.83)	344(13.6)	139(5.5)	2047(80.9)	
Middle	1094(22.41)	121(11.1)	45(4.1)	928(84.8)	
Rich	1257(25.75)	129(10.3)	35(2.8)	1093(87.0)	

Table 1. (Continued)

Characteristics	Overall[a] N (%)	Wasting		Nourished, N (%)	Chi-square value [df]
		Moderate, N (%)	Severe, N (%)		
Toilet facilities					13.52 [6]**
No facilities	162(3.32)	31(19.1)	10(6.2)	121(74.7)	
Hanging toilet	197(4.04)	28(14.2)	7(3.6)	162(82.2)	
Pit toilet	4173(85.49)	498(11.9)	192(4.6)	3483(83.5)	
Flush toilet	349(7.15)	37(10.6)	10(2.9)	302(86.5)	
Division					23.29 [12]**
Barisal	591(12.11)	85(14.4)	36(6.1)	470(79.5)	
Chittagong	912(18.68)	111(12.2)	46(5.0)	755(82.8)	
Rajshahi	617(12.64)	90(14.6)	29(4.7)	498(80.7)	
Rangpur	657(13.46)	84(12.8)	31(4.7)	542(82.5)	
Sylhet	842(17.25)	88(10.5)	32(3.8)	722(85.7)	
Khulna	521(10.67)	57(10.9)	25(4.8)	439(84.3)	
Dhaka	741(15.18)	79(10.7)	20(2.7)	642(86.6)	

[1]Data is presented as number (percentages).

df; degrees of freedom.

[a]Total number of children may differ because of missing data.

* denotes significant at 10% level; ** denotes significant at 5% level; *** denotes significant at 1% level.

Table 2. Multinomial logistic regression analysis for moderate and severe wasting in rural Bangladesh

Characteristics	Moderate Wasting		Severe Wasting	
	OR [95% CI]	P-Value	OR [95% CI]	P-Value
Sex of child				
Male	1.12[0.95-1.34]	0.171	1.62[1.22-2.15]	0.001***
Female (ref.)				
Child age (months)				
0-11	1.22[0.89-1.66]	0.207	1.56[0.98-2.48]	0.058
12-21	0.97[0.75-1.25]	0.822	1.45[0.97-2.17]	0.065
22-34	0.87[0.68-1.11]	0.263	0.91[0.67-1.56]	0.915
35-59 (ref.)				
Size at birth				
<Average	1.61[1.24-2.08]	0.000***	1.71[1.18-2.48]	0.005***
≥Average (ref.)				
Measles vaccination in first 9 months				
No	0.80[0.61-1.04]	0.100	1.43[0.97-2.11]	0.065
Yes (ref.)				
Fever in 2 weeks				
No	0.86[0.72-1.03]	0.107	0.85[0.64-1.12]	0.250
Yes (ref.)				

Characteristics	**Moderate Wasting**		**Severe Wasting**	
	OR [95% CI]	**P-Value**	**OR [95% CI]**	**P-Value**
Diarrhea in 2 weeks				
No	0.74[0.52-1.07]	0.113	0.75[0.43-1.29]	0.301
Yes (ref.)				
Maternal BMI (kg/m2)				
≤ 18.50	1.71[1.18-2.48]	0.005***	1.41[1.04-1.90]	0.025**
>18.50 (ref.)				
Maternal height (cm)				
<145	1.28[1.00-1.62]	0.044**	1,07[0.73-1.58]	0.713
≥145 (ref.)				
Mother's exposure to television				
No	1.07[0.83-1.39]	0.555	1.15[0.76-1.76]	0.504
Yes (ref.)				
Wealth index				
Poor	1.17[0.88-1.58]	0.275	1.69[1.04-2.77]	0.038**
Middle	1.00[0.75-1.33]	0.995	1.29[0.80-2.11]	0.302
Rich (ref.)				
Toilet facilities				
No facilities	1.44[0.81-2.56]	0.204	1.10[0.41-2.95]	0.836
Hanging toilet	1.00[0.56-1.77]	0.999	0.59[0.21-1.68]	0.325
Pit toilet	0.92[0.62-1.35]	0.673	0.96[0.47-1.95]	0.926
Flush toilet (ref.)				
Division				
Barisal	1.45[1.03-2.02]	0.030**	2.30[1.30-4.06]	0.004***
Chittagong	1.21[0.89-1.65]	0.219	2.03[1.18-3.49]	0.010**
Rajshahi	1.45[1.06-2.02]	0.026**	1.83[1.02-3.31]	0.043**
Rangpur	1.19[0.85-1.68]	0.294	1.78[0.99-3.20]	0.053
Sylhet	0.91[0.65-1.27]	0.599	1.26[0.71-2.26]	0.425
Khulna	1.13[0.78-1.64]	0.491	1.96[1.06-3.60]	0.030**
Dhaka (ref.)				

Reference Category: Nourished; ref: Reference; OR: Odds ratio; CI: Confidence interval.

** denotes significant at 5% level; *** denotes significant at 1% level.

DISCUSSION

In spite of having admirable success in fulfilling MDGs to reduce child and maternal mortality, the 2014 BDHS data revealed that nearly fifteen percent of total under five years old children in Bangladesh were acute malnourished (wasting) where 16.7% rural and 13% urban children were wasted. This study was set out to examine the associated factors of acute malnutrition (i.e., WHZ < -2, which comprises both moderate and severe wasting) among rural Bangladeshi children aged under five years old. After controlling the variables multinomial logistic regression analysis found that a range of variables such as sex of child, size at birth, mother's BMI (kg/m2), mother's height (cm), wealth index and division are responsible for wasting in rural children.

Being male has found as a risk factor of child wasting which is consistent with previous studies where male gender were more prone to be acutely malnourished. Bangladeshi rural male children were 1.62 times more likely to be severely wasted than those of their counterparts. Similar results also found in studies conducted in different countries [24, 34–37]. Generally, it was established that in south Asia the female children are more deprived of having basic needs and they treated unevenly. But this result is worth pointing out to announce that the situation is changing. Female are getting more attention to family due to government and NGOs initiatives. Already, the government of Bangladesh inserted various programs and policies to bring female children under mainstreaming that are helping out female from being suffering of malnutrition.

Children size at birth had an impact of wasting in both moderate and severe forms. The children who had less than average birth size were at more prone to be moderately and severely wasted than those children who were perceived as good size at birth by their mothers. This finding is in line with the previous findings where smaller birth size was associated with wasting [34-35, 38-39]. This could be because of mother's lack of nutrition which is also strongly associated with lower size babies [40], and unlimately contributing to acute malnutrition. As a lower birth size is significantly associated with wasting necessary measures need to be taken for improving the maternal nutritional capacity so that they can give birth of health baby. In Bangladesh, there is enough room remains to change the nutritional capacity of the rural mother. For example, rural mothers are living in a more vulnerable situation because of their socio-economic conditions. Therefore, current study recommends special attention to develop interventions like – free of medical care and nutritional food supply should be given to rural mothers. Additionally, community clinic should be modernized with adequate facilities and practitioners so that they can give service to the rural mothers in any emergency.

Finding of the study has signaled that low maternal health condition i.e., low BMI of mother has a negative impact on wasting of children. Mother's BMI is an independent risk factor for wasting/acute malnutrition. The prevalence of wasting observed to be increased with low mother's BMI. Mother's having with low BMI (<18.50 kg/m2) ran 1.71 and 1.41 times more likelihood to be wasted in both moderate and severe categories. Our study broadly supports those of the previous studies reported that low BMI is responsible for acute malnutrition of children aged under five years old [16-17, 25, 27, 29, 34, 36, 38]. As mother's BMI is an outcome of nutrition so there is no way of ignoring mother's nutritional status in formulating and inserting any programs or policies. Also rural mothers are not so aware of their nutritional status so an initiative needs to be taken to make then conscious about nutrition, health foods intake, and health outcomes, etc. In addition, findings of the current study show that maternal short stature and wasting are linked with each other which is in consistent with other studies [41–43].

As predicted, wealth index was closely linked with acute malnutrition which is similar to the previous done studies [10, 30, 41, 44]. This may be possibly due to the fact that wealth is the precondition for standard of living. A richer family can buy nutritional foods for its mothers, and even can arrange adequate medical checkup during the pregnancy. If any problems related to mother's health arise, rich household can take immediate cure so in later the mother get birth a healthier baby. In Bangladesh, the rural people are generally poor. They are often unable to intake nutritional foods during pregnancy even after the delivery of baby. So, this system put them into a vicious cycle of malnutrition. Therefore, to make any policies to improve the socio-economic status of the rural family could be a good mechanism to improve child health in Bangladesh.

Regional differences have been identified as a significant risk factor for childhood malnutrition. Finding exerts that compared to the children of Dhaka division, the children of both Barisal division and Rajshahi division were found to be at a higher risk of being moderately and severely wasted.

Several studies have documented region as a significant predictor for childhood acute malnutrition [3, 17, 34]. In this point of view, this study recommends that regional inequalities should be removed through special care of socioeconomic policies implementation.

There has been some deterioration in child nutritional status over the past decade (see, Figure 1). In 2000, the wasting among rural Bangladeshis children was about 11.6%. However, over the years it has been seeing an increasing trend and it has increased 14.5 % to 19.7% in 2007. The wasting rate has slightly decreased since 2007, and remained fairly constant at about 16.4% between 2011 and 2014 surveys.

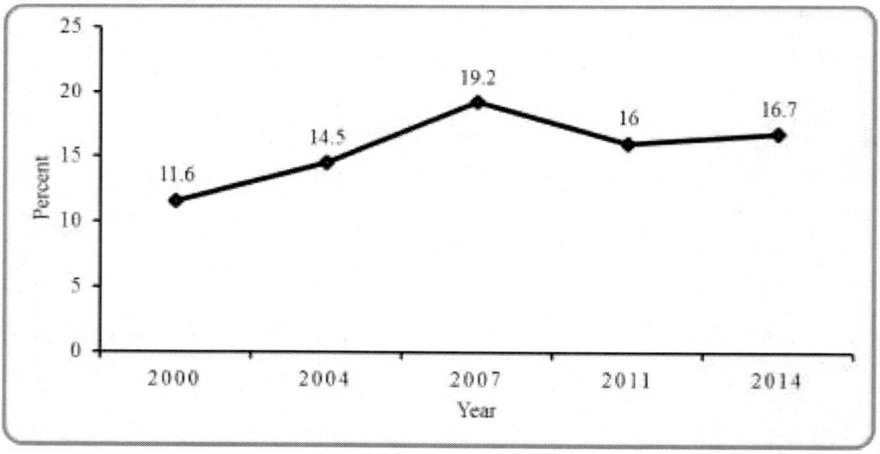

Figure 1. Extent of wasting among Bangladeshis rural children over the years.

LIMITATIONS

The first important limitations of this study is its cross-sectional nature, that didn't allows us to state the identified associated factors as definite causally related factors. For instances, some information like food intake of the mother during pregnancy, breastfeeding information, gestation period, mothers infection had not included in the survey which may be affect the findings. However, despite having limitations, appropriate care has been taken to interpret the findings in line with previous literature. Consequently this significant research would be an addition in literature to understand the child acute malnutrition in other poor developing countries across the world.

CONCLUSION

This study examined the factors which are responsible for childhood malnutrition among rural Bangladeshi children aged under five years old. Findings revealed that socioeconomic and biological factors are profoundly linked with childhood wasting, especially in rural children in Bangladesh. Nevertheless, most of the significant factors identified in this research are amendable by taking organized efforts and interventions. As the prevalence of wasting is still very high, there is no way of ignoring this problem. Therefore, to diminish the burden of malnutrition among children, a combined effort by the government, NGOs and the community are just needed to improve the nutritional status of the children along with mothers' health. Regarding to improve the entire nutritional capacity government may wish to design intervention programs/strategies by targeting the vulnerable groups of people in the society such as female and children. Finally, access to health information through all-kinds of media are to be engaged with rural community. Also health education content to be included from the primary level education system in the country.

ACKNOWLEDGMENTS

The authors are grateful to the National Institute of Population Research and Training (NIPORT), Bangladesh for providing the BDHS, 2014 data for public usage. Authors are also acknowledged to the reviewers for their effective and valuable comments.

FUNDING

Not applicable.

COMPETING INTERESTS

The authors declare that they have no competing interests.

ETHICAL CONSIDERATION

This study was based on analysis of an existing survey data obtained from Bangladesh Demographic and Health Survey, 2014 that was collected by means of a joint effort of NIPORT, ICF International (USA) and Mitra and Associates. The survey was approved by the Ethics Committee in Bangladesh and the Ethics Committee of the Demographic and Health Surveys (DHS) Programs. We were granted use of the data for independent research purposes.

REFERENCES

[1] Andaleeb, S. S., Siddiqui, N., Khandakar, S.: Patient satisfaction with health services in Bangladesh. *Health policy and planning, 22(4),* 263-273 (2007). doi: 10.1093/heapol/czm017.

[2] Ahsan, K. Z., Streatfield, P. K., Ijdi, R. E., Escudero, G. M., Khan, A. W., Reza, M. M.: Fifteen years of sector-wide approach (SWAp) in Bangladesh health sector: an assessment of progress. *Health policy and planning*, *31*(5), 612-623 (2015). doi: 10.1093/heapol/czv108.

[3] Chowdhury, S., Banu, L. A., Chowdhury, T. A., Rubayet, S., Khatoon, S.: Achieving millennium development goals 4 and 5 in Bangladesh. *BJOG: An International Journal of Obstetrics &*

Gynaecology, *118*, 36-46 (2011). doi: 10.1111/j.1471-0528.2011.03111.x.

[4] Rahman, A., Chowdhury, S.: Determinants of chronic malnutrition among preschool children in Bangladesh. *Journal of biosocial science*, *39*(2), 161-173 (2007). doi:10.1017/S0021932006001295.

[5] Black, R. E., Victora, C. G., Walker, S. P., Bhutta, Z. A., Christian, P., De Onis, M., Uauy, R.: Maternal and child undernutrition and overweight in low-income and middle-income countries. *The lancet*, *382*(9890), 427-451 (2013). doi:10.1016/S0140-6736(13)60937-X.

[6] Alom, J., Quddus, M. A., Islam, M. A.: Nutritional status of under-five children in Bangladesh: a multilevel analysis. *Journal of biosocial science*, *44*(5), 525-535 (2012). doi: 10.1017/S0021932012000181.

[7] Rahman, A., Rahman, M. S.: Rural-Urban Differentials of Childhood Malnutrition in Bangladesh. *International Journal of Child Health and Nutrition*, *8*(1), 35-42 (2019). doi: 10.6000/1929-4247.2019.08.01.5.

[8] Demissie, S., Worku, A.: Magnitude and factors associated with malnutrition in children 6-59 months of age in pastoral community of Dollo Ado district, Somali region, Ethiopia. *Sci J Public Health*, *1*(4), 175-83 (2013). doi: 10.11648/j.sjph.20130104.12.

[9] Pravana, N. K., Piryani, S., Chaurasiya, S. P., Kawan, R., Thapa, R. K., Shrestha, S.: Determinants of severe acute malnutrition among children under 5 years of age in Nepal: a community-based case–control study. *BMJ open*, *7*(8), e017084 (2017). http://dx.doi.org/10.1136/bmjopen-2017-017084.

[10] Meshram, I. I., Arlappa, N., Balakrishna, N., Rao, K. M., Laxmaiah, A., Brahmam, G. N. V.: Trends in the prevalence of undernutrition, nutrient & food intake and predictors of undernutrition among under five year tribal children in India. *Asia Pacific journal of clinical nutrition*, *21*(4), 568-576 (2012). http://dx.doi.org/10.6133%2fapjcn.2012.21.4.12.

[11] Das, S., Rahman, A., Ahamed, A., Rahman, S. T.: Multi-level models can benefit from minimizing higher-order variations: An illustration

using child malnutrition data. *Journal of Statistical Computation and Simulation 89(*6): 1090-1110 (2019).

[12] Khanam, R., Nghiem, H. S., Rahman, M. M.: The impact of childhood malnutrition on schooling: evidence from Bangladesh. *Journal of biosocial science*, *43*(4), 437-451 (2011). doi: 10.1017/S0021932011000149.

[13] Pelletier, D. L., & Frongillo, E. A.: Changes in child survival are strongly associated with changes in malnutrition in developing countries. *The Journal of nutrition*, *133*(1), 107-119 (2003). doi: 10.1093/jn/133.1.107.

[14] Skrable, K., Bilal, S., Sharma, R., Robertson, S., Ashenafi, Y., Nasrin, S., Levine, A. C.: The Effects of Malnutrition and Diarrhea Type on the Accuracy of Clinical Signs of Dehydration in Children under Five: A Prospective Cohort Study in Bangladesh. *The American journal of tropical medicine and hygiene*, *97*(5), 1345-1354 (2017). doi: 10.4269/ajtmh.17-0277.

[15] Mohsena, M., Goto, R., Mascie-Taylor, C. N.: Socioeconomic and demographic variation in nutritional status of under-five Bangladeshi children and trend over the twelve-year period 1996–2007. *Journal of biosocial science*, *49*(2), 222-238 (2017). doi: 10.1017/S002193201 6000328.

[16] Rahman, A.: "Estimating small area health-related characteristics of populations: A methodological review." *Geospatial Health 12(*1): 3-14 (2017).

[17] Das, S., Gulshan, J.: Different forms of malnutrition among under five children in Bangladesh: a cross sectional study on prevalence and determinants. *BMC Nutrition*, *3*(1), 1 (2017). doi: 10.1186/s40795-016-0122-2.

[18] Rahman, A., Rahman, M. S., Rahman, M. A.: Determinants of Infant Mortality in Bangladesh: A Nationally Surveyed Data Analysis: Determinants of Infant Mortality in Bangladesh. *International Journal of Child Health and Nutrition*, *8*(3) (2019).

[19] World Health Organization, & Unicef.: WHO child growth standards and the identification of severe acute malnutrition in infants and

children: joint statement by the World Health Organization and the United Nations Children's Fund (2009).

[20] Collins, S., Dent, N., Binns, P., Bahwere, P., Sadler, K., Hallam, A.: Management of severe acute malnutrition in children. *The lancet, 368*(9551), 1992-2000 (2006). doi: 10.1016/S0140-6736(06)69443-9.

[21] Kaiser, R., Chakauya, J. M., Shibeshi, M. E., of the Inter-country, E. U., for East, S. T., Africa, S., for Africa, R. O.: Trends in differences between births and surviving infants reported for immunization program planning and external data sources in Eastern and Southern Africa 2000–2013. *Vaccine, 34*(9), 1148-1151 (2016). doi: 10.1016/j.vaccine.2015.05.074.

[22] de Onis, M., Brown, D., Blossner, M., Borghi, E.: Levels and trends in child malnutrition. joint child malnutrition estimates. Technical report, UNICEF Geneva and WHO Washington DC and World Bank, 2015 (2015).

[23] Babatunde, R. O., Olagunju, F. I., Fakayode, S. B., Sola-Ojo, F. E.: Prevalence and determinants of malnutrition among under-five children of farming households in Kwara State, Nigeria. *Journal of Agricultural Science, 3*(3), 173-181 (2011).

[24] Rabbi, A. M. F., & Karmaker, S. C.: Determinants of child malnutrition in Bangladesh-A multivariate approach. *Asian journal of medical sciences, 6*(2), 85-90 (2015). doi: 10.3126/ajms.v6i2.10404.

[25] Rahman, A., Chowdhury, S., Hossain, D.: Acute malnutrition in Bangladeshi children: levels and determinants. *Asia Pacific Journal of Public Health, 21*(3), 294-302 (2009). doi: 10.1177%2F1010 539509335399.

[26] Alom, J., Islam, M. A., Quddus, M.: Socioeconomic factors influencing nutritional status of under-five children of Agrarian families in Bangladesh: A multilevel analysis. *Bangladesh Journal of Agricultural Economics, 32*(454-2016-36445), 63-74 (2009).

[27] Rayhan, M. I., Khan, M. S. H.: Factors causing malnutrition among under five children in Bangladesh. *Pak J Nutr, 5*(6), 558-62 (2006).

[28] Rahman, M. S., Howlader, T., Masud, M. S., Rahman, M. L.: Association of low-birth weight with malnutrition in children under

five years in Bangladesh: do mother's education, socio-economic status, and birth interval matter? *PloS one*, *11*(6), e0157814 (2016). doi: 10.1371/journal.pone.0157814.

[29] Rahman, M. M.: Is Unwanted birth associated with child malnutrition in Bangladesh? *International perspectives on sexual and reproductive health*, *41*(2), 80-88 (2015). doi: 10.1363/4108015.

[30] Musa, M. K., Muhammad, F., Lawal, K. M., Chowdhury, A. A., Hossain, A.: Risk factors of severe acute malnutrition among under-five children: a hospital-based study in Bangladesh. *J Med Sci Health*, *3*, 13-21 (2017).

[31] Oninla, S. O., Owa, J. A., Onayade, A. A., Taiwo, O.: Comparative study of nutritional status of urban and rural Nigerian school children. *Journal of tropical pediatrics*, *53*(1), 39-43 (2006). doi: 10.1093/tropej/fml051.

[32] Van de Poel, E., O'Donnell, O., Van Doorslaer, E.: Are urban children really healthier? Evidence from 47 developing countries. *Social science & medicine*, *65*(10), 1986-2003 (2007). doi: 10.1016/j.socscimed.2007.06.032.

[33] National Institute of Population Research and Training - NIPORT/Bangladesh, Mitra and Associates/Bangladesh, and ICF International. *Bangladesh Demographic and Health Survey 2014.* Dhaka: NIPORT, Mitra and Associates, and ICF International, (2016).

[34] Akombi, B. J., Agho, K. E., Hall, J. J., Merom, D., Astell-Burt, T., Renzaho, A. M.: Stunting and severe stunting among children under-5 years in Nigeria: A multilevel analysis. *BMC pediatrics*, *17*(1), 15 (2017). doi: 10.1186/s12887-016-0770-z.

[35] Megabiaw, B., Rahman, A.: Prevalence and determinants of chronic malnutrition among under-5 children in Ethiopia. *International Journal of Child Health and Nutrition*, *3*(2): 230-236 (2013).

[36] Asfaw, M., Wondaferash, M., Taha, M., Dube, L.: Prevalence of undernutrition and associated factors among children aged between six to fifty nine months in Bule Hora district, South Ethiopia. *BMC Public health*, *15*(1), 41 (2015). doi: 10.1186/s12889-015-1370-9.

[37] Khan, G. N., Turab, A., Khan, M. I., Rizvi, A., Shaheen, F., Ullah, A., Ariff, S.: Prevalence and associated factors of malnutrition among children under-five years in Sindh, Pakistan: a cross-sectional study. *BMC nutrition*, *2*(1), 69 (2016). doi: 10.1186/s40795-016-0112-4.

[38] Islam, M. M., Marium, U.: Small size at birth as a predictor of increased risk of childhood morbidity, mortality and malnutrition: Evidence from Bangladesh demographic and health survey. *Journal of Biostatistics and Epidemiology*, *4*(2), 33-44 (2018).

[39] Aheto, J. M. K., Keegan, T. J., Taylor, B. M., Diggle, P. J.: Childhood Malnutrition and Its Determinants among Under-Five Children in G hana. *Paediatric and perinatal epidemiology*, *29*(6), 552-561 (2015). doi: 10.1111/ppe.12222.

[40] Rahman, A., Harding, A.: *Small area estimation and microsimulation modeling*. Boca Raton, USA: CRC Press, (2017).

[41] Ambadekar, N. N., Zodpey, S. P.: Risk factors for severe acute malnutrition in under-five children: a case-control study in a rural part of India. *Public Health*, *142*, 136-143 (2017). doi: 10.1016/j.puhe.2016.07.018.

[42] Özaltin, E., Hill, K., Subramanian, S. V.: Association of maternal stature with offspring mortality, underweight, and stunting in low-to middle-income countries. *Jama*, *303*(15), 1507-1516 (2010). doi: 10.1001/jama.2010.450.

[43] Martorell, R., Young, M. F.: Patterns of stunting and wasting: potential explanatory factors. *Advances in Nutrition*, *3*(2), 227-233 (2012). doi: 10.3945/an.111.001107.

[44] Fakir, A. M., Khan, M. W. R.: Determinants of malnutrition among urban slum children in Bangladesh. *Health economics review*, *5*(1), 22 (2015). doi: 10.1186/s13561-015-0059-1.

In: Malnutrition
Editor: Azizur Rahman

ISBN: 978-1-53617-597-4

Chapter 4

AN ELL TYPE SMALL AREA ESTIMATION APPROACH FOR BINARY RESPONSE VARIABLE WITH APPLICATION TO BANGLADESH CHILD MALNUTRITION STUDY

Sumonkanti Das*[*], *Abdullah Al Islam, Bappi Kumar, Luthful Alahi Kawsar and Zakir Hossain, MD
Department of Statistics, Shahjalal University of Science & Technology, Sylhet, Bangladesh

ABSTRACT

Now-a-days governments and policy makers focus more on public health indicators at disaggregated level administrative units. The World Bank small area estimation (SAE) method known as ELL method has been widely used for estimating poverty and child malnutrition at micro-level administrative units for many developing countries using continuous response variables like household expenditure and children height-for-age Z-score (HAZ). However, health indicators like diarrhoea

[*] Corresponding Author's Email. sumonkanti-sta@sust.edu.

prevalence are based on categorical attributes and hence the ELL method cannot be implemented directly. The idea of ELL approach can be implemented after developing a generalized linear mixed model for the categorical response variable. An ELL type SAE approach has been proposed for binary response variable and evaluated through simulation studies and an empirical study using children HAZ data extracted from Bangladesh Demographic and Health Survey 2011 and the 5% of 2011 Census data. District level estimates of stunting (HAZ < -2.00) and severe stunting (HAZ < -3.00) are calculated considering both continuous and binary response variables for examining the performance of the proposed SAE method. Findings of both simulation and empirical studies reveal feasibility of the SAE method for binary response variable.

Keywords: height-for-age Z-score, stunting, severe stunting, World Bank method

INTRODUCTION

Small area estimation (SAE) is a statistical technique to obtain estimates with better precision for the desired disaggregated level administrative units of a large population such as a country [1]. The basic idea of SAE method is to combine a survey data with a recent census or administrative data via a statistical model [2] or spatial model [3-5]. It requires both survey data consisting of target variable and the associated explanatory variables, and census data consisting of all the explanatory variables specified in the regression model. The most important note is that the SAE method is based on model-based approach, where response values are assumed to follow a super-population model and uncertainty comes from model misspecification, instead of design-based approach, where response values are assumed fixed and uncertainty comes from sampling errors [6].

The World Bank has been utilising an SAE method known as ELL method after the authors Elbers, Lanjouw, and Lanjouw [7] for poverty and nutrition mapping in many developing countries including Bangladesh. The basic idea of the ELL methodology is to develop a regression model of a continuous response variable (such as per capita consumption expenditure, height-for-age Z-score) on some explanatory variables common in both survey and census data at least by definition. When the variable of interest is categorical more commonlly binary such as incidence of diarrhoea (a child has experienced with diarrhoea or not during a fixed time period preceding the survey) instead of continuous, the ELL methodology cannot be implemented directly. The basic idea of the ELL method can be implemented after developing a generalized linear mixed model (GLMM) more specifically a logistic random effects model for the dichotomous response variable [8-12]. The main difficulty is to develop a proper GLMM model incorporating the available survey data with a recent census or administrative data for a country. Also the development process varies over countries due to survey and census data structure as well as complexity in modelling when the occurance of event is rare like diarrhoea and acute respiratory infection (ARI) among under five years of children.

In small area estimation of child malnutrition, a continuous response variable say height-for-age Z-score (HAZ) is modelled based on the survey data and then HAZ score is predicted for all census children using the census values of the explanatory variables. The ultimate parameters such as proportion of stunted (hereafter S2) and severely stunted (hereafter S3) children using the cut-offs HAZ < -2.00 SD and HAZ < -3.00 SD respectively along with their precisions are obtained via a suitable bootstrap procedure based on the same developed model of HAZ. However, it is not possible to have such continuous variable for public health indicators like prevalence of diarrhoea, fever, anemia, and ARI which are usually categorical (preferably dichotomous) variables. Also, if the continuous HAZ score is not available but children nutrition status is available only, then we have to utilize an alternative SAE technique based on generalized mixed model using the nutrition status. So, an SAE idea following the approach of ELL method is required to develop for dichotomous response variable. In this study an attempt has been made to propose an ELL type SAE approach for the dichotomous type response variable. The simplicity and wide application of the ELL method to developing countries like Bangladesh are the main reason of considering ELL type SAE method among the other competent SAE methods like empirical best prediction (EBP) [13] and M-quantile (MQ) [14] methods. A recent study [15] on the comparison of ELL, EBP and MQ also stimulates enthusiasm to focus on ELL type SAE estimator for binary response variable

The main objective of this study is to develop an SAE method for dichotomous response variable following the ELL approach and then implement the method to the child malnutrition data of Bangladesh. To examine the performance of the developed SAE method, both model-based and design-based simulation studies have been conducted at first and then the proposed idea is empirically evaluated by estimating the proportion of stunting and severe stunting children at division and district levels in Bangladesh through the application of the existing ELL method to the HAZ variable and the proposed SAE method to nutrition status of stunting and severe stunting.

The remainder of this Chapter is organized as follows. Section 2 (Data and Methods) briefly describes survey and census data used in this study, the standard ELL method for continuous response, and the proposed ELL type SAE method for binary response. The procedures and results of the design- and model-based simulation studies are illustrated in Section 3 (Simulation Studies). The empirical results obtained from Bangladesh child malnutrition study are demonstrated in Section 4 (Application to Bangladesh Child Nutrition Study). The Chapter concludes with summary of the numerical and empirical evalauation of the proposed SAE method in the Conclusion Section.

DATA AND METHODS

Data

In this study, Bangladesh Demographic and Health Survey (BDHS) 2011 and a 5% sample of Bangladesh Population and Housing Census data have been utlized for simulation and empirical studies. These data sets are briefly described below.

Bangladesh Population and Housing Census (BPHC) 2011

Bangladesh is divided into a total of 7 divisions for administrative determinations. The lower administrative units are zila (district), upazila (sub-district), union/ward, and Mauza. These lower administrative units are not generally considered in the sampling design of any nationwide household survey of Bangladesh. The lowest unit considered for sampling design in different surveys is the enumeration area (EA), which can be a village, part of village or combination of several villages.

The full census data of Bangladesh is huge and also not available for academic purposes. However, 5% of the full census data is available from BBS. The 5% sample of the full census is selected via a systematic random sampling method with sampling interval, k = 20 where household (HH) is the sampling unit. The 5% census dataset consists of 7,205,720 individuals from 1,609,088 HHs covering all administrative units up to sub-district level. This sample census consists of 15,93,096 General HHs covering all administrative units up to sub-district level. A total of 751,906 under-5 children are found in these general HHs based on which the ultimate parameters of this study are estimated. Mean number of children at district level in the census sample is 11749 with a minimum of 2504 children.

The census data cover information on some important socio-demographic characteristics including age, sex, education, schooling, employment, disability and housing characteristics. Contextual variables at district and sub-district level are generated from the 5% census data and utilized in model specification. Some key indicators at different population hierarchy (e.g., population density at sub-district level) available from BBS website (based on full census) are also used in model construction.

Bangladesh Demographic and Health Survey (BDHS) 2011

Demographic and health related data have been collecting in Bangladesh by Demographic and Health Surveys (DHS) program since 1993-94. The sampling design of BDHS 2011 is based on concurrent Census 2011 - which is the main reason for considering BDHS 2011 instead of recent 2014 BDHS. The BDHS 2011 is conducted following a two-stage stratified sampling design (20 strata, 600 EAs, 30 households per

EAs) covering all divisions and districts. The completed data have 17141 households, 17842 ever-married women aged 12-49 years, and 8753 under-5 children [16]. Anthropometric nutrition data were available for a total of 7647 children. Mean number of children at district level is 137 with a minimum of 15 children in the survey data. Out of 546 sub-districts, only 396 are covered in the BDHS 2011. The full hierarchy form children to division (children-HH-Cluster-Upzila-Zila-Division) has been created by merging different DHS data sets which are freely avaiable from DHS website (www.dhsprogram.com).

Methods

Children anthropometric index HAZ is utilized as continuous response variable to validate the proposed SAE method. A child is determined as stunted (lower height compared to age) if HAZ< -2.00 standard deviation (SD) otherwise not stunted. In this report, the continuous response variable is denoted by Y and then the corresponding binary response variable by Z.

Suppose y_{ijk} is the HAZ score for k^{th} child belongs to j^{th} household (HH) of ith cluster. It is assumed that the anthropometric index follows either a 2-level or 3-level superpopulation model as

$$y_{ijk} = \mathbf{x}_{ijk}^T \beta + u_{ij} + \varepsilon_{ijk} \text{ or } y_{ijk} = \mathbf{x}_{ijk}^T \beta + \eta_i + u_{ij} + \varepsilon_{ijk}$$

where $\mathbf{x}_{ijk}^T$ is a vector of explanatory information, β is the vector of regression parameters and η_i, u_{ij} and ε_{ijk} are respectively cluster, HH, and child-specific random errors. It is assumed that the level-specific random errors are identically and independently distributed with mean zero and homoskedastic error variances $\hat{\sigma}^2_{\eta(l)}$, $\hat{\sigma}^2_{u(l)}$, and $\hat{\sigma}^2_{\varepsilon(l)}$ respectively where the suffix (l) for $l-$ level model. Assuming normality of the level-specific random errors, the models can be developed following standard maximum likelihood (ML) or restricted ML (REML) method. The fitted models can be used to estimate mean and distribution functions (say, HAZ < t) of a nutrition index at different hierarchies (as for example, division and district in this study).

We note that the auxiliary variables may be useful primarily in explaining the cluster-level variation, or the household-level variation. If variation at a particular level is explained more by a model, the respective error variance will be smaller. The estimate for a particular small area will typically be the average of the predicted y_{ijk}s in that area. Because the standard error of a mean gets smaller as the sample size gets bigger, the contribution to the overall standard error of the variation at each level depends on the sample size at that level. The number of households in a small area will typically be much larger than the number of clusters, and the number of children under-5 larger again, so to get small standard errors for the small area estimates it is of particular importance that, at the highest level, the unexplained cluster-level variance $\hat{\sigma}^2_{\eta(l)}$ should be small. Two important diagnostics of the model-fitting stage, in which the relationship between Y and X is estimated for the survey data, are the R^2 measuring how much of the variability in Y is explained by X, and the ratio $\hat{\sigma}^2_{\eta(3)} \big/ \left(\hat{\sigma}^2_{\eta(3)} + \hat{\sigma}^2_{u(3)} + \hat{\sigma}^2_{\varepsilon(3)}\right)$ measuring how much of the unexplained variation is at the cluster level.

Design-Based Direct Estimator

The Horvitz-Thompson estimator for estimating mean and total of a super-population in a stratified sample can be utilized to obtain design-based direct estimates of target parameter for small areas using the response values available in the survey data. The design-based direct estimator (denoted by DIR) for the target proportion P_i for area i is

$$\hat{P}_i^{DIR} = \sum_{j \in s_i} w_{ij} z_{ij}, i = 1, \ldots, D$$

where z_{ijk} is either 1 (stunted child) or 0 (not stunted child) and $w_{ij} = w^*_{ij} \big/ \sum_{j \in s_i} w^*_{ij}$ is normalized survey weights for unit (children) j in area (say, district) i with $\sum_{j\in s_i} w_{ij} = 1$ and w_{ij}^* is survey weight (inverse of the inclusion probability) for unit j in area i. The design-based variance of the direct estimator $\hat{P}_i^{Dir}$ can be approximated following Särndal et al. [17].

The direct survey estimator is unbiased but becomes inefficient when area specific sample size is small. The confidence interval for the direct estimates are also very large due to high design-based variance of direct estimator. Further, for areas with no sample data, direct estimates cannot be used (for example, many subdistricts have no sample information in BDHS 2011 data). Thus, direct estimates are discouraged for the small areas. In this context model-based SAE methods that 'borrow strength' via statistical models can be used to produce reliable small area estimates. These methods typically involve the use of indirect estimators based on suitable linking model [18].

ELL Method for Continuous Response Variable

In this study, the World Bank SAE method for continuous response variable is used instead of other SAE methods like EBP and MQ methods. The ELL procedure is sub-divided into two stages: fitting regression model at first and then prediction of the response variable for all census units based on the fitted model. After fitting the regression model and obtaining the corresponding parameters, the second stage of the ELL method is to conduct either a parametric bootstrap (PB) or a non-parametric bootstrap (NPB) procedure to obtain the area-specific poverty estimates of interest and their corresponding estimated mean square errors (ESMEs) [7, 19]. For both the PB or NPB procedures the basic steps are:

- Step 1: generate regression parameters $\boldsymbol{\beta}^*$ from a suitable sampling distribution, say the multivariate normal distribution $N\left(\hat{\boldsymbol{\beta}}_{gls}, \hat{\mathbf{v}}\left(\hat{\boldsymbol{\beta}}_{gls}\right)\right)$;
- Step 2: generate level-specific random errors using an appropriate parametric distribution or by resampling via simple random

sampling with replacement (SRSWR) from the estimated level-specific sample residuals;

- Step 3: generate bootstrap response values y_{ijk}^{*} using the generated regression parameters and the level-specific random errors. The generated response values are used to estimate the area-specific parameter of interest say $P_i^{*} = N_i^{-1}\sum_{j=1}^{C_i}\sum_{k=1}^{N_{ij}} I\left[y_{ijk}^{*} < t\right]$ for a specific value of t (say, here $t =$ -2.00).

These three steps are iterated for a large number of times say B = 500 and then the mean and variance of these B estimates are considered as the final estimates and their MSEs respectively as

$$\hat{P}_i^{ELL} = B^{-1}\sum_{b=1}^{B} P_i^{*} \text{ and } se_i^{ELL} = B^{-1}\sum_{b=1}^{B}\left(P_i^{*} - \hat{P}_i^{ELL}\right)^2 .$$

This estimator is denoted by ELL.C in the text since the proportion of stunting is calculated based on the ELL approach for continuous response variable.

Proposed ELL Type Method for Binary Response Variable

For explaining the small area statistical methodology for dichotomous response variable (say, stunting), let the child-level measurement z_{ijk} is either 1 (stunted child) or 0 (not stunted child) and $p_{ijk} = \text{prob}\left(z_{ijk} = 1\right)$ represents the probability of being stunted for k^{th} child belonging to j^{th} household of ith cluster (EA in census data). As ELL methodology, the first target is to develop a nested-error logistic regression model of z_{ijk} as below:

$$\text{logit}\left(p_{ijk} \mid \mathbf{X}_{ijk}, \eta_i, u_{ij}\right) = \log\left[p_{ijk} / \left(1 - p_{ijk}\right)\right] = \mathbf{X}_{ijk}^{T}\boldsymbol{\beta} + \eta_i + u_{ij}$$

Or

$$\text{logit}\left(p_{ijk} \mid \mathbf{X}_{ijk}, u_{ij}\right) = \log\left[p_{ijk} / \left(1 - p_{ijk}\right)\right] = \mathbf{X}_{ijk}^{T}\boldsymbol{\beta} + u_{ij}$$

where $\mathbf{X}_{ijk}$ is vector of explanatory information, $\boldsymbol{\beta}$ is vector of regression parameters, the terms η_i , and u_{ij} corresponds to cluster and household specific random errors respectively. The random errors are usually assumed independent and identically distributed with mean zero and homoskedastic error variances $\hat{\sigma}^2_{\eta(l)}$ and $\hat{\sigma}^2_{u(l)}$. The considered random intercept logistic regression model (denoted by GLMM) can be fitted by estimating regression parameters and variance components [18]. The regression model can be extended to higher level, however the ELL methodology assumes heterogeneity at cluster-level rather than higher levels [7]. The small area estimates and their mean squared error (MSE) can be calculated via either a parametric or semi-parametric bootstrap procedure. In each bootstrap, response values P^*_{ijk} are predicted for all census children by generating regression parameters and level-specific errors from their parametric (or empirical) distributions. The estimates at target level are obtained by aggregating P^*_{ijk} belong to the corresponding level. The bootstrap procedure is done for B = 500 times and then the ultimate parameters with their MSEs are calculated by taking average and variance of B estimates respectively. The steps can be illustrated as the aforementioned steps for the continuous response variable as:

- Step 1: fit random effects logistic model to obtain regression coefficients with their estimated variance-covariance matrix and variance components.
- Step 2: generate regression parameters $\boldsymbol{\beta}^*$ from a suitable sampling distribution, say the multivariate normal distribution $N\left(\hat{\boldsymbol{\beta}}_{gls}, \hat{\mathbf{v}}\left(\hat{\boldsymbol{\beta}}_{gls}\right)\right)$;
- Step 3: generate level-specific random errors (except the children level) using an appropriate parametric distribution or by

resampling via simple random sampling with replacement (SRSWR) from the estimated level-specific sample residuals;

- Step 4: generate bootstrap response values p_{ijk}^{*} using the generated regression parameters and the level-specific random errors. The generated response values are used to estimate the area-specific parameter of interest say $P_i^* = N_i^{-1}\sum_{j=1}^{C_i}\sum_{k=1}^{N_{ij}} p_{ijk}^{*}$.

The steps 2-4 are iterated for a large number of times say $B = 500$ and then the mean and variance of these B estimates are considered as the final estimates and their MSEs respectively as

$$\hat{P}_i^{ELL} = B^{-1}\sum_{b=1}^{B} P_i^* \text{ and } se_i^{ELL} = B^{-1}\sum_{b=1}^{B}\left(P_i^* - \hat{P}_i^{ELL}\right)^2.$$

This estimator is denoted by ELL.B in the text since the estimator is developed based on the traditional ELL approach but used for binary response variable.

SIMULATION STUDIES

The numerical evaluation of the proposed SAE approach for binary response has been done through both design-based and model-based simulation studies. For both these simulation studies, the child nutrition data of BDHS is considered as the census data, i.e., a finite population which consists of response values for a fixed number of children. In design-based simulation study, the response values are assumed constant while in the model-based simulation study the response values are assumed to follow a super-population model. For conducting the simulation studies, the districts (only 64) are considered as clusters and divisions (only 7) are considered as target small area so that proper sample can be drawn following different complex design.

In the simulation study, the HAZ score is considered as the continuous response variable and nutrition status based on HAZ (Z = 0 if HAZ < -2.00, otherwise Z = 1) is considered as binary response variable. The reason of choosing two-types of variables is to show how the ELL approach can be implemented for both continuous and binary response variable under two-types of simulation studies. It is assumed that if the ELL approach for binary response perform very similar to the established ELL approach for continuous response, the proposed approach can be considered reasonable to implement in the SAE study using real dichotomous data like diarrhoea and ARI prevalance.

Here the finite population consists of D = 7 small areas (divisions), C = 64 clusters (districts) and 7467 children. The real clusters (primary sampling units) are not considered in the simulation due to very small size of clusters (ranges 1-20 children per cluster). The districts are considered as clusters since the minimum number of children was found 15 and hence a sample can be drawn from each cluster. Since the survey data consists of 7647 (here N) children, approximately 10% of the total children is considered as the sample. For simplicity, n = 7*110 = 770 children are aimed to select in the sample. However, different sampling procedures have been considered to prepare different scenarios to conduct the simulation studies.

Scenarios Based on Survey Sampling Design

In the simulation studies, six different scenarios are prepared based on six different sampling procedure mainly various types of simple random sampling (SRS) and cluster random sampling (CRS) methods. Since we need all the target areas (division here) to cover in the sample, the same sampling procedure has been conducted for each of the areas. The scenarios are as below:

- *Scenario 1* (SRS with equal number of children per area): From each division, equal number of children are selected randomly without consideration of area size.
- *Scenario 2* (SRS with proportional allocation of children): The number of sampled children are considered based on the number of children per division, i.e.,the larger sub-population, the larger the sub-sample. However, the selection of children are not dependent on the cluster (district here).
- *Scenario 3* (SRS with Optimum (Neyman) allocation of children): Here the number of children are considered based on area-specific variation in the response variable, i.e., the higher the variation in HAZ score, the larger the number of children per area. Thus, the children HAZ score is consider as the design-variable to draw the sample. It is noted that, the selection of children is still not dependent on the cluster.
- *Scenario 4* (Two-stage CRS with equal allocation of cluster): In this case, 28 clusters (out of 64 districts) are considered to select covering all the 7 areas. Since minimum number of districts per division is 4, 4 districts are randomly selected from each division at the first stage in this scenario. In the second stage, the district-specific number of children are sampled proportional to the selected district-specific total number of children.
- *Scenario 5* (Two-stage CRS with proportional allocation of cluster): In this case, the number of (28 out of 64 districts) are considered following probability proportional to size covering all the 7 areas. The higher the number of clusters of an area might have higher chance of having more clusters. Then the children from the selected clusters are randomly selected as in Scenario 4.
- *Scenario 6 (*Two-stage CRS with Optimum (Neyman) allocation of cluster): In this scenario, the number of clusters is selected based on area-specific variation of HAZ variable, i.e., the higher the variation in HAZ, the higher the chance of selecting clusters. Then the children are randomly selected from the selected areas as per

scenarios 4 and 5. The sampling designs of these scenarios are briefly illustrated in Table 1.

In each scenario, three estimators DIR (Horvitz-Thompson estimator), ELL.C and ELL.B are applied to estimate proportion of stunting at division level with their mean squared. To conduct the study, the scenarios are repeated for S = 500 times each with B = 500 bootstraps. In the simulation study, performance of the indicator estimator only (not its standard error estimator) is assessed. The ELL estimator is expected to provide very small RMSE (and hence poor coverage rate) since the cluster-level variability is found insignificant in most of the samples drawn from the study.

Table 1. Scenarios of simulation study based on stratified simple random sampling (SRS) and Cluster Random Sampling (CRS) designs

Scenario	Type of sampling design	Distribution of children	Number of stages	Distribution of clusters
1	Stratified SRS	Equal	1	Unequal
2	Stratified SRS	Proportional	1	Unequal
3	Stratified SRS	Optimal	1	Unequal
4	Stratified CRS	Unequal	2	Equal
5	Stratified CRS	Unequal	2	Proportional
6	Stratified CRS	Unequal	2	Optimal

The relative bias (RB), and relative root mean squared errors (RRMSE) are considered as the performance measure of the direct and SAE estimators. The mean of RBs and RRMSEs over areas are calculated to compare the DIR, ELL.C and ELL.B estimators. The RB and RRMSE are calculated as below

$$RB_i = P_i^{-1} \times S^{-1}\sum_{s=1}^{S}\left(\hat{P}_i^{(s)} - P_i^{(s)}\right) \text{ and } RRMSE_i = P_i^{-1} \times \sqrt{S^{-1}\sum_{s=1}^{S}\left(\hat{P}_i^{(s)} - P_i^{(s)}\right)^2}$$

where $P_i = S^{-1}\sum_{s=1}^{S} P_i^{(s)}$ is the average proportion for area i over S = 500 simulations.

Results from Design-Based Simulation Study

The mean relative bias (RB, %) and relative root mean squared errors (RRMSE, %) over areas for the considered estimators are shown in Table 2 for all scenarios. Both the ELL.C and ELL.B estimators are providing design-bias estimates while the DIR estimator provides design-unbiased estimates as expected. However, DIR estimators provides very inconsistent results due to comparatively lower sample size per area. In terms of both RB and RRMSE, the ELL.C is performing slightly better than the ELL.B estimators, though ELL.B follows the trend of the results of ELL.C. The correlations of the estimated proportions of stunting by the ELL.B and ELL.C estimators shown in Table 3 indicate that they are highly positively correlated in all the scenarios. Though the correlations for the estimated stunting are very high (more than 0.90) and do not vary much by the scenarios, the correlations for the estimated RMSEs vary over scenarios: higher than 0.60 for the SRS scenarios and around 0.70 for the CRS scenarios.

Table 2. Average of estimated Relative Bias (RB, %) and Relative Root Mean Squared Errors (RRMSE, %) over small areas for the direct (DIR), ELL estimators for continuous (ELL.C) and binary (ELL.B) responses under the considered scenarios under design-based simulation study

Scenarios	RB (%)			RRMSE (%)		
	DIR	ELL.C	ELL.B	DIR	ELL.C	ELL.B
1	0.91	1.38	1.19	7.32	2.23	2.86
2	-0.06	1.04	0.93	7.61	2.28	3.06
3	-0.24	0.86	0.84	7.68	2.37	3.05
4	1.17	1.46	1.58	8.61	2.53	3.13
5	1.05	1.70	1.73	9.22	2.91	3.38
6	0.54	1.50	1.59	9.12	3.06	3.40

Table 3. Correlation between ELL.C and ELL.B estimators according to scenarios under design-based simulation study

	Correlations					
Scenarios	**1**	**2**	**3**	**4**	**5**	**6**
Estimate Proportion	0.94	0.92	0.92	0.93	0.93	0.93
Estimated RMSE	0.61	0.62	0.63	0.74	0.71	0.68

Results from Model-Based Simulation Study

In the model-based simulation, the dependent variable is assumed to follow a super-population model with 2-level assuming children as level-1 and district as level-2 following the ELL approach. The level-specific random errors are assumed to follow normal distribution with mean zero and variances respectively $\hat{\sigma}_u^2 = 0.02$ and $\hat{\sigma}_\varepsilon^2 = 1.66$ respectively. The regression coefficients of the considered super-population model of HAZ given in Appendix Table 1, which is based on the real survey data of child malnutrition. The estimated variance-covariance matrix of the estimated regression coefficients are also given in Appendix Table 2. The values of explanatory variables are remained same in each of the simulation procedure and the corresponding regression coefficients are generated from multivariate normal distribution with mean vector $\hat{\beta}$ and variance-covariance matrix $\text{cov}\left(\hat{\beta}\right)$. After generating response values for each of the population units, a random sample is chosen as per the sampling design explained in Table 1 and then the small area target parameters are estimated. The simulation procedure is repeated for S = 500 times for each of the six scenarios.

The mean relative bias (RB, %) and relative root mean squared errors (RRMSE, %) over areas for the considered estimators are shown in Table 4 for the all scenarios under model-based simulation study. In terms of RB, the DIR estimator followed by ELL.B estimator performs better than the ELL.C estimator, however both ELL.C and ELL.B provides lower RRMSE than DIR estimator. Under the complex sampling designs 4-6 (stratified CRS), ELL.B outperforms than the DIR estimator in terms of both RB and RRMSE. The correlations of the estimated proportions of stunting by the ELL.B and ELL.C estimators shown in Table 5 indicate that they are highly positively correlated (about r = 0.95) in all the scenarios. The correlations for estimated RMSE are also found highly positive (around 0.80). It is also noted that the RRMSEs increase with the complexity of the sampling design in both types of simulation studies.

Table 4. Average of estimated Relative Bias (RB, %) and Relative Root Mean Squared Errors (RRMSE, %) over small areas for the direct (DIR), ELL estimators for continuous (ELL.C) and binary (ELL.B) response variables under model-based simulations

Scenarios	**RB (%)**			**RRMSE (%)**		
	DIR	**ELL.C**	**ELL.B**	**DIR**	**ELL.C**	**ELL.B**
1	0.47	-0.67	0.18	7.44	5.89	6.35
2	0.14	-0.35	0.36	7.78	6.04	6.53
3	-0.06	-0.49	0.25	7.64	5.93	6.42
4	0.86	-0.49	0.35	9.08	6.12	6.55
5	0.65	-0.31	0.43	9.52	6.33	6.92
6	-0.24	-0.67	0.01	9.93	6.45	6.98

Table 5. Correlation between the estimates and their estimated RMSE by the ELL.C and ELL.B estimators according to scenarios under model-based simulations

	Correlations					
Scenarios	1	2	3	4	5	6
Estimate Proportion	0.96	0.96	0.96	0.96	0.96	0.96
Estimated RMSE	0.84	0.81	0.83	0.79	0.84	0.80

The main target of the simulation studies is to show how the ELL estimator for binary response work compared to the ELL estimator for continuous response in estimating proportion of children HAZ< -2.0 SD. The results from both types of simulation studies support that the ELL.B performs very similar to the ELL.C estimator, even in the complex sampling design ELL.B outperform the ELL.C under model-based simulation. The important note is that, the RB under model-based simulation are comparatively lower than those under design-based studies. The main reason is that the random effects are remained fixed under the design-based simulation, while the random effect tends to zero over simulation. In design-based simulation, the ELL estimators would perform better in terms of bias if the area-variability can be captured by including more explanatory variables, which is the practice in the ELL method implementation [19]. The provision of including as much as possible explanatory variables is due to account for the variability of the response variable at higher administrative level. If the variability cannot be capture in the model, the ELL estimator provides higher bias and lower mean squared errors due to ignorance of area-variability [20]. As a consequence, the ELL estimator provides lower coverage rate of the true parameters.

APPLICATION TO BANGLADESH CHILD NUTRITION STUDY

To evaluate how the proposed SAE idea for binary response does perform in a real data, an attempt has been made here to estimate district level child undernutrition in Bangladesh using the continuous response variable HAZ as well as a binary response variable (Stunted: HAZ < -2.0, Not Stunted: HAZ ≥ -2.0) following the World Bank SAE approach. The study utilized 2011 BDHS, and the 5% of 2011 Census data. It is assumed that if both the SAE approaches behave similarly, then the proposed SAE idea for binary response can be considered reasonable for implementation.

The World Bank SAE method (ELL approach) for poverty mapping has been utilized for estimating child nutrition indicators (stunting, wasting and underweight) using the three different anthropometric indices including HAZ [21, 22]. In the ELL method, a single developed model of HAZ can be used to determine the proportion of stunted (hereafter S2) and severely stunted (hereafter S3) children using the cut-offs HAZ < -2.00 SD and HAZ < -3.00 SD respectively. The SAE estimates for S3 are expected to be relatively less precise than those of S2, since the number of children with HAZ < -3.00 SD is smaller than the number of children with HAZ < -2.00 SD. When the continuous HAZ variable is not available but children nutrition status is available only, then the proposed SAE method based on logistic mixed model for each of the nutrition indicators can be utilized following the existing ELL approach. To evaluate the performance of the proposed method, S3 and S2 estimates at district level are calculated by developing (i) a linear mixed model of HAZ for implementing the existing ELL method for continuous response and (ii) two logistic models for S2 and S3 separately for implementing the proposed ELL type method for binary response.

Multilevel Models

Several 2-level and 3-level models are developed considering children, HH, cluster, and sub-district as the consecutive hierarchies for the HAZ. The summary statistics of the fitted models shown in Table 6 indicate that the sub-district specific 3-level model (denoted hereafter 3L.HH.SD) perform slightly well than the cluster-specific 3-level model (denoted by 3L.HH.CL) in terms of conditional AIC (cAIC), R^2, and likelihood ratio test (LRT). The 3L.HH.CL model also behave similar to the 3L.HH.SD, but since the mean cluster size in the census data is very small (only 3), this model is not used for prediction purpose. Additionally, about 42% sub-districts have only single cluster, which suggest: (i) cluster and sub-district specific variance components can be difficult to estimate simultaneously and (ii) either cluster or sub-district specific model can be equivalently used. Thus, the 3L.HH.SD model is chosen for implementing the ELL method for continuous response. As a diagnostic of the selected 3L.HH.SD model, the Q-Q plots of the estimated level-specific residuals are plotted in Figure 1, which reveals that all the residuals are approximately normally distributed. The fitted model is given in the Appendix Table 3.

Table 6. Summary statistics of the fitted multilevel models for Height-for-age Z-score (HAZ)

Model	df	Random-effects Parameters			Margi-nal R^2	Conditi-onal R^2	BIC	cAIC
		σ_η^2	σ_u^2	σ_ϵ^2				
2L.HH	20	-	0.3461	1.3688	13.68	31.10	25925	25569.82
2L.CL	20	0.0591	-	1.6565	13.26	16.25	25942	25761.79
3L.HH.CL	21	0.0529	0.3012	1.3621	13.42	31.28	25903	25517.58
3L.HH.SD	21	0.0478	0.3067	1.3618	13.64	31.48	25892	25505.75
LR test of H_0: $\sigma_\eta^2 = 0$: χ^2 = 30.881, P-value = 0.000 (3L.HH.CL vs. 2L.HH).								
LR test of H_0: $\sigma_\eta^2 = 0$: χ^2 = 41.795, P-value = 0.000 (3L.HH.SD vs. 2L.HH)								

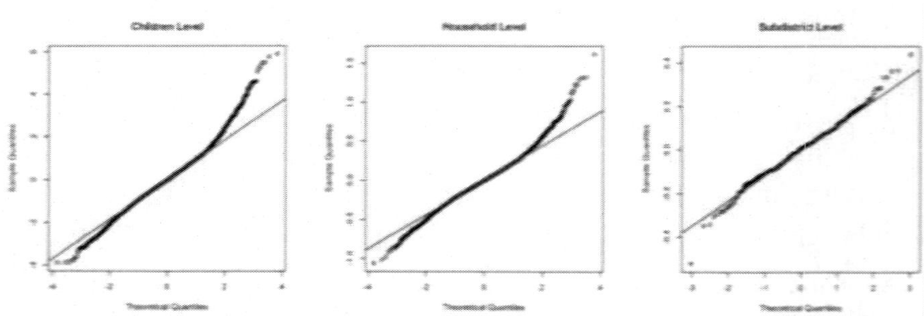

Figure 1. Q-Q plots of the level-specific residuals for the fitted 3-level model of HAZ.

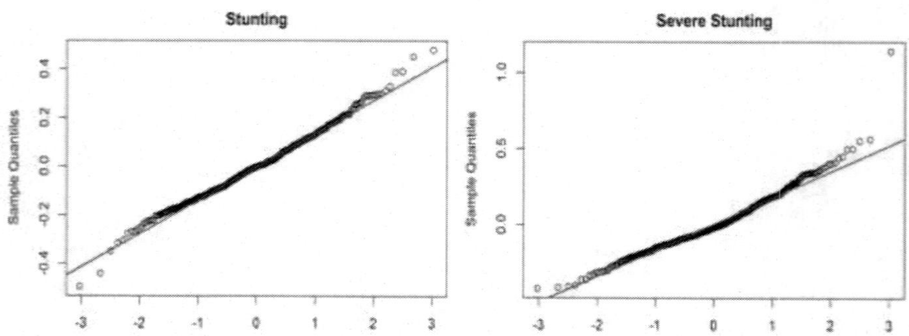

Figure 2. Q-Q plots of the Sub-district level residuals obtained from logistic mixed model for stunting (S2) and severe stunting (S3).

Table 7. Summary statistics of the fitted multilevel models for Stunting (S2) and Severe Stunting (S3)

Nutrition Indicator	Model	DF	Parameter (σ_u^2)	Marginal R^2	Conditional R^2	BIC
Stunting	2L.SD	19	0.0813	14.34	16.41	9652.8
Severe Stunting	2L.SD	17	0.1502	14.93	18.65	6171.9

In case of S2 and S3, 2-level logistic models considering children and sub-district (denoted by 2L.SD) as the two consecutive levels are developed. A number of attempts have been made to accommodate the HH as an intermediate level for constructing a 3-level model, but the corresponding HH-level variance component behaves differently from that of the HAZ model. Mainly the additive property of the variance components does not exist and so HH is ignored in model development. Thus, we used 2L.SD model instead of restrict ourselves to utilize a 3-level model for the proposed SAE method of dichotomous response. The summary statistics of the fitted models for S2 and S3 are shown in Table 7. The regression coefficients of these two models are given respectively in Appendix Table 4 and Appendix Table 5. As diagnostics of the two models for S2 and S3, Q-Q plots of the sub-district specific estimated random effects shown in Figure 2 confirm their normality. Hereafter, the SAE estimators based on continuous and dichotomous response variables are denoted by ELL.C and ELL.B respectively.The estimators are compared with the design-based direct estimator denoted by DIR.

Stunting and Severe Stunting at Division and District Levels

The proportion of stunting (S2) and severe stunting (S3) at division level estimated by the DIR, ELL.C, and ELL.B estimators are shown in Table 8. Theoretically, the DIR estimator is design-unbiased at both national and division level. Table 8 shows that the ELL estimators provide estimates very similar to the DIR estimator at both levels, though the ELL.B estimator provides slightly higher RMSE. Table 8 also reveals that the ELL.B estimator behaves similar to the direct estimator in case of S3 as well as its RMSE. Though the ELL.C provides comparatively lower RMSE for S3, it provides slightly higher proportion of S2 and S3 than those of the DIR and ELL.B estimators.

When turn to the district level estimates, both the ELL estimators perform significantly better than the DIR estimator in each case of S2 and S3 in terms of RMSE. The comparison of the ELL estimates with the direct estimates shown in Figure 3 indicates that the ELL.B seems closer to the diagonal line, which indicates that the ELL.B may provide slightly more unbiased estimates than ELL.C. This tendency is more obvious in case of S3. To examine the performance of the RMSE estimator, the estimated RMSEs are plotted against the number of children per district in Figure 4.

Table 8. Division level estimates of S2 and S3 with their standard errors (RMSEs) using DIR, ELL.C and ELL.B estimators

Division	Stunting			Sever Stunting		
	Prevalence (%)					
	DIR	ELL.C	*ELL.B*	DIR	ELL.C	*ELL.B*
Barisal	44.24	43.72	*43.38*	19.90	18.71	*16.51*
Chittagong	40.87	42.46	*42.69*	15.71	18.09	*16.55*
Dhaka	42.90	42.48	*43.87*	15.12	18.05	*16.32*
Khulna	33.42	38.57	*37.07*	10.69	15.58	*12.35*
Rajshahi	33.51	36.38	*34.81*	8.74	14.14	*8.92*
Rangpur	42.47	45.65	*45.88*	15.92	19.99	*17.97*
Sylhet	49.62	51.30	*52.65*	22.19	24.71	*24.78*
Bangladesh	40.40	42.55	*42.84*	15.20	18.18	*16.03*
	RMSE × 100					
Barisal	2.44	1.46	*1.49*	1.96	1.01	*1.22*
Chittagong	1.18	0.97	*1.08*	0.87	0.66	*0.87*
Dhaka	1.01	0.99	*1.10*	0.73	0.66	*0.85*
Khulna	1.75	1.77	*2.08*	1.15	1.13	*1.48*
Rajshahi	1.52	1.62	*2.01*	0.91	1.06	*1.15*
Rangpur	1.71	1.21	*1.38*	1.27	0.94	*1.05*
Sylhet	2.06	1.75	*2.17*	1.71	1.45	*2.13*
Bangladesh	0.56	0.68	*0.79*	0.41	0.49	*0.60*

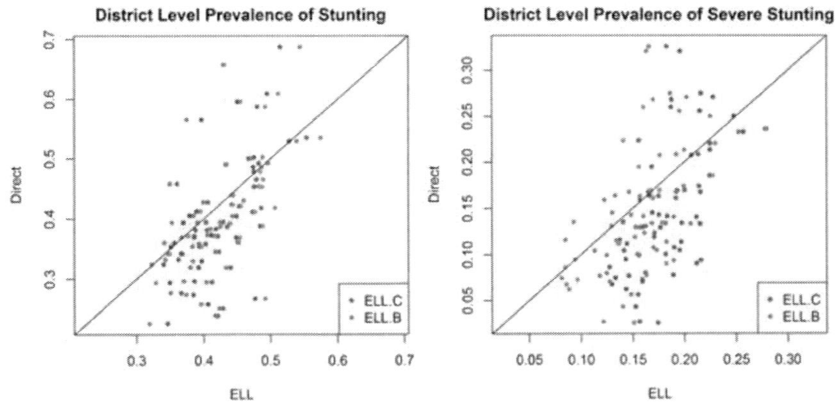

Figure 3. ELL-based estimates (ELL.C & ELL.B) against direct estimates (Direct) of stunting (S2) and severe stunting (S3).

The figure clearly shows that ELL.C performs slightly better than the ELL.B in terms of RMSE. However, the performance of the ELL.B estimator seems very similar to the ELL.C in case of both estimates and RMSE. The performance between these two estimators is not directly comparable due to difference in response type, explanatory variables, fitted multilevel models and the estimation method. The basic difference may also be due to omitting the HH level in fitting the multilevel logistic model.

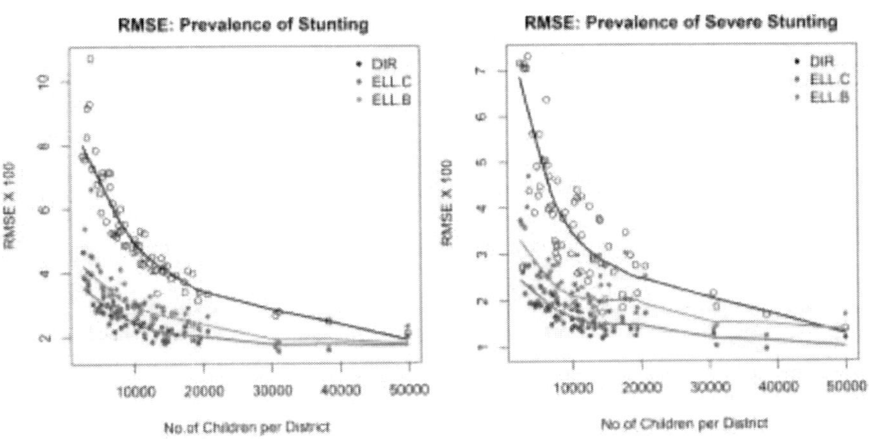

Figure 4. Estimated root mean squared error (RMSE) of stunting (S2) and severe stunting (S3) using direct (DIR) and ELL-based estimates (ELL.C & ELL.B) against the district-specific number of under-5 children.

CONCLUSION

A small area estimation technique for binary response variable has been developed by adapting the SAE approach of World Bank known as ELL method for estimating poverty indicators at disaggregated administrative units using a continuous response variable such as household per capita expenditure/income. Then the developed SAE idea has been applied to children nutrition data of Bangladesh for estimating proportion of stunted and severaly stunted children at district and sub-district levels. The proposed SAE method has been evaluated through design- and model-based simulation studies considering various complex sampling designs and through an empirical validation study. Child nutrition data of BDHS 2011 have been utilized in simulation studies as well as for empirical validation study.

In the simulation studies, the continuous anthropometric HAZ score and the child nutrition status have been used as the continuous and binary response variables respectively to apply the ELL type SAE estimator for continuous (ELL.C) and binary (ELL.B) response variables. The simulation studies show that the ELL.B performs better than the ELL.C estimator in terms of RB, while ELL.C provides slightly lower RRMSE. Even in case of more complex sampling design, the ELL.B tends to be more unbiased than the design-based direct estimator. Thus it can be said that the ELL.B may tend to be more unbiased but less consistent than the ELL.C estimator under the considered scenarios. Overall, both the ELL.B and ELL.C estimators perform very similar in all the scenarios with some exception of RB.

In the empirical validation study, the ELL.B and ELL.C estimators are applied to estimate district level stunting and severe stunting. In both cases, the ELL.B is found more unbiased than the ELL.C in comparison to the direct (DIR) estimator, which actually reveals the results of model-based simulation study. In terms of RMSE, the ELL.C provides slightly lower RMSE than does ELL.B, which may be the effect of failure to include household in the model as an intermediate level. Though household level explanatory variables are included in the model, still the ELL.C estimator is based on a powerful model than that of the ELL.B estimator. The performance of ELL.B for stunting and severe stunting confirms that the estimator can be utilized at different cut-off points (or tails of a distribution). Thus findings of the simulation studies and the empirical validation studies support that the proposed SAE method for binary response variable performs in the line of the existing World Bank SAE method for continuous response.

There are still more investigations are required for examining the performance of the proposed SAE estimator for binary response variable. Simulation studies are required to examine how the SAE method is robust to model misspecification (either violation of distribution of random errors or ignorance of any important level of the underlying superpopulation model) and outliers. In this study, the small areas are assumed to have some sample observation in the simulation and empirical studies, and so it is still unknown how the method behaves for the non-sampled small areas. The proportion of stunting at sub-district level could be done in the simulation studies to examine how the estimator behave. Since appropriate sampling procedure cannot be made with the survey data structure of BDHS 2011, the proportions at sub-district levels were not considered in the simulation studies. In future study, this can be done if a survey data support such simulation study.

As the standard ELLmethod, the proposed method may also have the problem of shrinkage to the population mean (if area-level variation cannot be captured by the model) and so possible approach may be required to unshrinkage the small area estimates following Carpenter, Goldstein, and Rasbash [23]. Further simulation works are required also for understanding the behavior of the SAE estimator with varying intra-cluster correlation (though the ELL method emphasizes more contextual variables in the model to minimize the intra-cluster correlation). More importantly, investigation of the MSE estimator based on the ELL type approach is still remained. The issues related to MSE estimation under violation of underlying assumptions can be brought in future studies following the related studies on the standard ELL methods [20, 24-25]. The problem of ignoring any important level of the superpopulation model can be solved by incorporating contextual variables (either calculating from unit-level census data or collecting from administrative/census report) in the model to account aggregated and disaggregated level variations, specifically sub-district, district and division levels in Bangladesh study [9].

In addition to basic modelling diagnostics of the SAE approach, the sensitivity of the proposed SAE method can be examined for different cut of points of the continuous response variable (say, HAZ < -3.0 SD, HAZ < -1.0 SD, HAZ > 2.0 SD). This examination might reveal how the proposed SAE method will behave for different types of indicators with higher or lower prevalence (as for example, proportion of pregnant women in Bangladesh who receive any antenatal care and who receive at least 4 antenatal cares). The stability of the SAE estimator might also vary with the cut-off points (i.e., the proportion of an event). Possible improvement of the proposed SAE estimator for binary response variable might help the demographers and policy makers to estimate public health indicators like diarrhoea, ARI, and anemia at disaggregated levels, which in turn help them in distributing aid to the vulnerable micro-level administrative hotspots.

ACKNOWLEDGEMENTS

The authors acknowledge Shahjalal University of Science & Technology University Research Center, Sylhet, Bangladesh and Ministry of Science & Technology, Government of Bangladesh, Dhaka, Bangladesh for funding the research work.

APPENDIX TABLES

Appendix Table 1. Fitted 2-level linear regression model for the considered Height-for-age Z-score (HAZ) variable

Variables	Estimate	Std. Error	df	t value	Pr(>|t|)
(Intercept)	-0.76974	0.067233	777.7192	-11.4489	3.71E-28
X1	0.064042	0.038227	6045.141	1.675312	0.093925
X2	-0.01362	0.000886	7608.459	-15.3766	1.44E-52
X3	-0.45921	0.037932	6130.576	-12.1062	2.35E-33
X4	-0.64507	0.087176	5489.861	-7.39964	1.57E-13
X5	-0.81362	0.132519	7635.202	-6.13966	8.68E-10
X6	0.212141	0.036551	7637.151	5.803935	6.74E-09
X7	0.141769	0.060065	55.75727	2.360241	0.021787
X8	-0.19885	0.093534	31.48333	-2.126	0.041445
$\hat{\sigma}_u^2$	0.02				
$\hat{\sigma}_\varepsilon^2$	1.80				
ICC	0.01				

Appendix Table 2. Estimated variance-covariance matrix (×100) of the estimated regression coefficients for the considered 2-level regression model of HAZ

Variables	(Intercept)	X1	X2	X3	X4	X5	X6	X7	X8
(Intercept)	0.45	-0.08	0.00	-0.11	-0.11	-0.51	-0.04	-0.14	-0.12
X1	-0.08	0.15	0.00	0.05	0.06	0.02	0.00	0.00	0.01
X2	0.00	0.00	0.00	0.00	0.00	0.00	0.00	0.00	0.00
X3	-0.11	0.05	0.00	0.14	0.11	-0.03	0.02	0.02	0.02
X4	-0.11	0.06	0.00	0.11	0.76	-0.08	0.02	0.03	0.00
X5	-0.51	0.02	0.00	-0.03	-0.08	1.76	-0.01	0.04	-0.02
X6	-0.04	0.00	0.00	0.02	0.02	-0.01	0.13	0.00	0.00
X7	-0.14	0.00	0.00	0.02	0.03	0.04	0.00	0.36	0.11
X8	-0.12	0.01	0.00	0.02	0.00	-0.02	0.00	0.11	0.87

Appendix Table 3. Random Intercept model for height-for-age Z-score (HAZ) for the under-5 children considering children at level-1, household (HH) at level 2, and sub-district at level-3, 2011 BDHS

Variables	Estimate	Std. Error	df	t value	Pr(>|t|)
(Intercept)	-1.26	0.14	1338.39	-9.03	0.00
Khu.Div	0.02	0.06	432.50	0.28	0.78
Raj.Div	0.24	0.06	402.05	4.01	0.00
Syl.Div	-0.19	0.07	240.96	-2.85	0.00
Urban	0.05	0.04	2486.96	1.11	0.26
age0	0.94	0.04	7171.37	24.43	0.00
age4	0.14	0.04	7180.61	3.81	0.00
pemp	-0.46	0.13	6402.28	-3.52	0.00
iwater_1	0.25	0.07	4837.31	3.37	0.00
ilattr_1	0.16	0.04	5803.84	4.56	0.00
ihtyp_2	-0.30	0.06	5870.95	-4.95	0.00
ihtyp_3	-0.59	0.06	5623.66	-9.36	0.00
ihtyp_4	-0.72	0.10	4759.33	-6.96	0.00
hedsec	0.18	0.04	6149.35	4.99	0.00
pkids06	-1.03	0.16	5557.38	-6.64	0.00
pkids714	-0.55	0.13	6523.52	-4.29	0.00
ptap_u_subdist	-0.46	0.14	959.70	-3.27	0.00
phhcssc_u_subdist	0.90	0.40	379.33	2.22	0.03

§ Descriptions of the variables are in Appendix Table 6

Appendix Table 4. Random Intercept logistic model for stunting (STUNT) for the under-5 children considering children at level-1, and sub-district at level-2, 2011 BDHS

Variable	Estimate	Std. Error	z value	Pr(>|z|)
(Intercept)	-0.56	0.20	-2.74	0.01
Khu.Div	-0.06	0.10	-0.56	0.58
Raj.Div	-0.39	0.09	-4.09	0.00
Syl.Div	0.22	0.10	2.31	0.02
Urban	-0.08	0.07	-1.15	0.25
age0	-1.33	0.07	-17.94	0.00
age4	-0.33	0.06	-5.34	0.00
pemp	0.40	0.20	1.99	0.05
iwater_1	-0.37	0.13	-2.91	0.00
ilattr_1	-0.24	0.06	-4.16	0.00
ihtyp_2	0.40	0.11	3.74	0.00
ihtyp_3	0.80	0.11	7.31	0.00
ihtyp_4	0.93	0.17	5.55	0.00
hedsec	-0.25	0.06	-4.02	0.00
pkids06	0.94	0.22	4.30	0.00
ptap_u_subdist	1.12	0.23	4.89	0.00
phhcssc_u_subdist	-1.69	0.61	-2.75	0.01
scale.pafem	-0.17	0.03	-6.54	0.00

Appendix Table 5. Random Intercept logistic model for severe stunting (SV.STUNT) for the under-5 children considering children at level-1, and sub-district at level-2, 2011 BDHS

Variable	Estimate	Std. Error	z value	Pr(>|z|)
(Intercept)	-2.44	0.20	-12.16	0.00
Khu.Div	-0.20	0.14	-1.45	0.15
Raj.Div	-0.73	0.15	-4.92	0.00
Syl.Div	0.40	0.12	3.47	0.00
Urban	0.03	0.10	0.30	0.76
age0	-1.17	0.11	-10.48	0.00
age4	-0.39	0.09	-4.61	0.00
ilattr_1	-0.40	0.08	-5.22	0.00
ihtyp_2	0.48	0.16	2.92	0.00
ihtyp_3	0.89	0.17	5.40	0.00
ihtyp_4	1.10	0.22	5.01	0.00
hedsec	-0.25	0.09	-2.80	0.01
pkids06	1.25	0.28	4.47	0.00
ptap_u_subdist	0.53	0.27	1.97	0.05
scale.pafem	-0.18	0.04	-5.07	0.00

Appendix Table 6. Description of response and explanatory variables used in model development

Name	Description	Type
HAZ	Height-for-age Z-score	Continuous
stunted	S2: HAZ < -2.00 SD	Indicator
Severe stunted	S3: HAZ < -3.00 SD	Indicator
Urban	Urban place of residence	Indicator
age0	Child age 0-11 month	Indicator
age1	Child age 12-23 month	Indicator
age4	Child age 48-59 month	Indicator
Chi.Div	Living in Chittagong division	Indicator
Khu.Div	Living in Khulna division	Indicator
Raj.Div	Living in Rajshahi division	Indicator
Syl.Div	Living in Sylhet division	Indicator
hedsec	Secondary educated household head	Indicator
iwater_1	Household's drinking water source: Tap	Indicator
ilattr_1	Household has sanitary latrine	Indicator
ihtyp_2	Household has Semi-pucka house	Indicator
ihtyp_3	Household has Katcha house	Indicator
ihtyp_4	Household has Jhupri house	Indicator
scale.pafem	Proportion of adult female member in household (Scaled)	Continuous
pkids06	Proportion of kids aged 0-6 year	Continuous
pkids714	Proportion of kids aged 7-14 years in household	Continuous
pemp	Proportion of employed family members in household	Continuous
ptap_u_subdist	Proportion of households with tap water at sub-district level	Continuous
phhcssc_u_subdist	Proportion of household head completed SSC at sub-district level	Continuous

References

[1] Rahman, A. (2017). Estimating small area health-related characteristics of populations: A methodological review. *Geospatial Health*, *12*(1), 3-14. [495]. https://doi.org/10.4081/gh.2017.495.

[2] Rao, J. (2003). *Small Area Estimation.* Hoboken, New Jersey: John Wiley & Sons, Inc.

[3] Rahman, A., & Harding, A. (2017). *Small area estimation and microsimulation modeling*. Boca Raton, USA: CRC Press. https://doi.org/10.1201/9781315372143.

[4] Rahman, A. (2017). Small area housing stress estimation in Australia: Calculating confidence intervals for a spatial microsimulation model. *Communications in Statistics Part B: Simulation and Computation*, *46*(9), 7466-7484. https://doi.org/10.1080/03610918.2016.1241406.

[5] Rahman, A., Harding, A., Tanton, R., & Liu, S. (2010). Methodological Issues in Spatial Microsimulation Modelling for Small Area Estimation. *International Journal of Microsimulation*, *3*(2), 3-22.

[6] Chambers, R., & Clark, R. (2012). *An introduction to model-based survey sampling with applications.* Oxford: Oxford University Press.

[7] Elbers, C., Lanjouw, J., & Lanjouw, P. (2003). Micro-Level Estimation of Poverty and Inequality. *Econometrica,* 71(1), 355–364.

[8] Haslett, S., Jones, G., Isidro, M., & Sefton, A. (2014). *Small Area Estimation of Food Insecurity and Undernutrition in Nepal.* Kathmandu: Central Bureau of Statistics, National Planning Commissions Secretariat, World Food Programme, UNICEF & World Bank.

[9] Das, S., Rahman, A., Ahamed, A., & Rahman, S. T. (2019). Multi-level models can benefit from minimizing higher-order variations: An illustration using child malnutrition data. *Journal of Statistical Computation and Simulation*, *89*(6), 1090-1110. https://doi.org/10.1080/00949655.2018.1553242.

[10] Das, S., Rahman, A., Kumar, B., Hossain, M. Z., & Rahman, S. T. (2019). Estimation of child under-nutrition at disaggregated administrative tiers of Sunamganj District in Bangladesh: An application of small area estimation method. In *Applied Statistics and Policy Analysis Conference, 2019: Effective policy through the use of big data, accurate estimates and modern computing tools and statistical modelling* (pp. 1). Springer.

[11] Yunus, R. M., & Rahman, A. (2018). Factors associated with nutritional status of children in low and middle income countries in Southeast Asia: A multilevel analysis. In P. Dalziel (Ed.), *Proceedings of the 42nd Annual Conference of the Australian & New Zealand Regional Science Association International (pp. 1-7). Australian & New Zealand Regional Science Association International (ANZRSAI)* (pp. 177-182). New Zealand: Agribusiness and Economics Research Unit.

[12] Ahamed, A., Das, S., Rahman, A., & Rahman, S. T. (2017). On Selection of a Robust Multilevel Model for Child Nutrition Measure in Bangladesh. In *Proceedings of the Bangladesh Statistical Association Conference 2017, Dhaka* (pp. 1-22).

[13] Molina, I., & Rao, J. N. (2010). Small area estimation of poverty indicators. Candian Journal of Statistics, 38(3), 369–385.

[14] Chambers, R., & Tzavidis, N. (2006). M-quantile models for small area estimation. *Biometrika,* 93(2), 255–268.

[15] Das, S., & Haslett, S. (2019). A Comparison of Methods for Poverty Estimation in Developing Countries. *International Statistical Review*, 87(2), 368-392.

[16] NIPORT, Mitra and Associates, & ICF International. (2013). *Bangladesh Demographic and Health Survey 2011.* Dhaka, Bangladesh and Calverton, Maryland, USA: National Institute of Population Research and Training (NIPORT), Mitra and Associates, and ICF International.

[17] Särndal, C. E., Swensson, B., & Wretman, J. (1992). *Model assisted survey sampling* (1st ed.). New York: Springer.

[18] Rao, J. N. K. & Molina, I. (2015). *Small Area Estimation.* Hoboken, New Jersey: John Wiley and Sons.

[19] Elbers, C., Lanjouw, J. O., & Lanjouw, P. (2002). Micro-level Estimation of Welfare. *World Bank Policy Research Working Papaer, 2911.* Washington DC: The World Bank.

[20] Das, S., & Chambers, R. (2017). Robust mean-squared error estimation for poverty estimates based on the method of Elbers, Lanjouw and Lanjouw. *Journal of the Royal Statistical Society: Series A (Statistics in Society)*, 180(4), 1137-1161.

[21] BBS & UNWFP (2004). *Local Estimation of Poverty and Malnutrition in Bangladesh.* Dhaka: Bangladesh Bureau of Statistics and United Nations World Food Programme.

[22] BBS, WFP, & IFAD (2014). *Small-Area Estimation of Child Undernutrition in Bangladesh.* Dhaka: Bangladesh Bureau of Statistics, World Food Programme and International Fund for Agricultural Development.

[23] Carpenter, J. R., Goldstein, H., & Rasbash, J. (2003). A novel bootstrap procedure for assessing the relationship between class size and achievement. *Journal of the Royal Statistical Society: Series C (Applied Statistics)*, 52(4), 431-443.

[24] Tarozzi, A. & Deaton, A. (2009). Using census and survey data to estimate poverty and inequality for small areas. *The Review of Economics and Statistics*, 91, 773–792.

[25] Das, S., Chandra, H., & Chambers, R. Robust Mean Squared Error Estimation for ELL-based Poverty Estimates under Heteroskedasticity - An Application to Poverty Estimation in Bangladesh. *Statistics and Applications*, 16(1), 2018, 375-397.

In: Malnutrition
Editor: Azizur Rahman

ISBN: 978-1-53617-597-4

Chapter 5

MALNUTRITION AND AGE-SPECIFIC CHILD MORTALITY BURDEN IN INDIA

*G. Naline**
Madras School of Economics, Chennai,
Tamil Nadu, India

ABSTRACT

Child survival is one of the prominent indicators of child health. Over one-third of all child deaths are linked to malnutrition. This paper examines the significance of socio- economic factors and intergenerational transmission factors associated with age specific mortality by using National Family Health Survey Data (NFHS-3). Cox proportional hazard models and life table techniques are used to determine the statistical significance of the variables used in the study. The results show that factors such as gender, birth order, birth interval and birth size have substantial effects on mortality. Girls of higher birth order survive more during the first month than boys and reverse is true where later born boys have survival advantage after the first month up to five years. Intergenerational transmission variables like mother's height,

* Corresponding Author's Email: naline@mse.ac.in.

weight, age of mother at first birth, diet patterns, and health seeking behavior are highly associated with all age specific mortality. There exists a strong association of domestic violence variable with neonatal mortality. Among the environmental features, the interaction term of open defecation with religion supports the findings from earlier studies that Muslim children have better survival advantage than their Hindu counterparts. This is due to the fact that open defecation is more in Hindu concentrated regions of rural areas and consequently the hazard ratios for Muslims are lower as of compared with Hindus. Short-term policies such as guidance and support for creating awareness on antenatal check-ups, institutional deliveries, longer birth intervals, shorter birth orders will help to curb the mortality of children.

Keywords: mortality, survival analysis, Cox proportional hazard models, malnutrition

INTRODUCTION

Malnutrition is a serious concern is highly ignored and unrevealed by the conventional reported child deaths. A child born and raised in an environment with adequate resources has a very low probability of mortality at a young age, is well nourished and grows up to live longer with a good standard of living. Malnutrition is one of the major factors related to child mortality which arises from numerable factors such as poor intake of nutrients [1, 2] poor environmental condition [3, 4] and inadequate access to public service programs and birth-related factors which lead to high levels of mortality. Therefore, it is of utmost priority to analyze the major consequence of malnutrition, child death. In health studies, child survival is a significant aspect which involves strategies and interventions to reduce child mortality. One of the targets on Millennium Development Goals (MDG) is to reduce under-five-year-old mortality by two thirds within 2015 which is popularly known as MDG 4 target. Since the era of MDG came to an end, the whole world community agreed on a new framework called the Sustainable Development Goals (SDGs), where the proposed target is within 2030. The main aim is to end preventable deaths of newborns and children under five years of age, where all countries aim to reduce neonatal mortality to at least as low as 12 deaths per 1,000 live births and under-five-year-old mortality to at least as low as 25 deaths per 1,000 live births.

Further, the chances of older children (2 to 5 years) getting affected when they have low weight and height to age where as malnutrition is the dominant cause of mortality among 0 to 5 year old children [5, 6]. Child survival continues to be a big priority since the recent UNICEF estimates predict that between 2019 and 2030, 52 million children under the age of five will die. [7]. Child mortality used to be very high in the earlier century across the globe. For example, in the 18th century, every third child died in Sweden. From 1990 to 2015, the trend shows a significant reduction in child mortality where, industrialized countries were able to reduce the child mortality to below 5 per 1000 live births because of the improvements in technology and awareness of health [8]. Failure to examine the pathways and links which causes mortality with its determinants will lead to incorrect policy decisions. Child mortality is often sensitive to socio-economic conditions of the economy in developing countries where due to economic crisis child mortality increased in Zimbabwe from 80 to 126 per 1000 live births whereas in developed countries, mortality is reduced due to technological improvements and improved cycles of fertility [9].

The next section discusses the gaps in literature arising from the determinants of childhood mortality rates from child, mother, household characteristics and interventions in India. The review also focuses on the modeling framework used to analyze mortality rates caused by these variables. Subsequent section presents the specific objectives, followed by a section that gives the description of the methodology of this study. The data and the study variables used in the econometric analysis are explained in the next section with preliminary graphs and tables. This is followed by a section providing the results of the estimated model and the last section gives the concluding remarks.

Child mortality refers to the death of children and infants. There are various types of child mortality depending on their period of survival. *Neonatal mortality* refers to the death of children within 28 days of life.

The probability of dying before the first birthday is known as *Infant mortality*. *Post neonatal mortality* refers to the difference between infant and neonatal mortality. If the child dies before the fifth birthday, it is commonly termed as *Under-five-year-old mortality*. And overall, the probability of the child dying between the 1st and the 5th birthday is expressed as *Child mortality*. In India, if we trace the trend of child mortality there is considerable amount of decline in the rates but the rate of decline is unsatisfactory. Major concern is on the neonatal mortality.

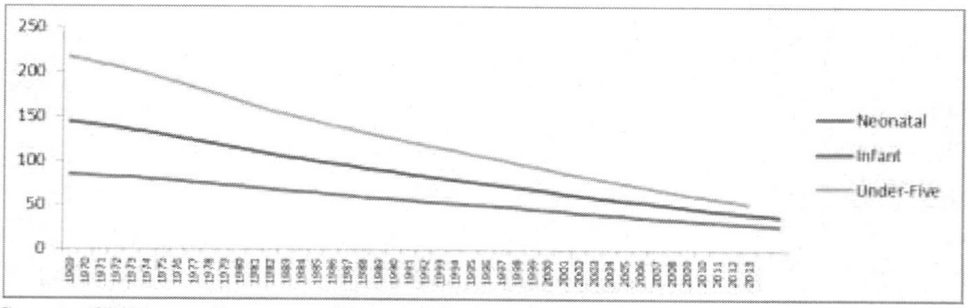

Source: Childmortality.org and Roser (2016).

Figure 1. Trends of mortality rates in India.

Figure 1 shows a declining trend in neonatal, infant and under-five-year-old mortality in India from 1969 to2013. In 1969, the rate was 86, 144 and 217 deaths per 1000 live births respectively and in 2013 it reduced to 52 deaths per 1000 live births. The fastest decline started from 1990 where the rates started to converge as well, but the rate of decline was not able to meet the MDG targets. In short, the rates are declining n India but it is less impressive than the poorer counterparts of other South and South- East Asian countries [10]. There are various causes of child mortality like household factors, environmental, social and demographic causes, birth related issues and health care utilization and access. It is imperative to identify the causes if the child mortality rates have to be reduced. At the macro level, [11] argues that reduction of childhood mortality increases the economic growth and in turn growth reduces mortality. Similarly, using Demographic Health Surveys (DHS) data for middle income countries, another paper identified that aggregate economic shocks increases infant mortality. For example, when Peru was in crisis during 1998 and 1990, the infant mortality increased from 61 to 72 per 1000 births [12].

The broad area of this research addresses the variations which causes a large gap between the mortality rates across various states in India. To understand the variations which cause inequalities, it is inevitable to identify the causes/determinants which are responsible for these variations. This study explores the covariate effects of child mortality on various determinants such as socio-economic factors of households, environmental characteristics at Primary Sampling Unit (PSU) level, health-seeking behavior and attitude of mothers and other determinants. Since most of the factors are correlated and interlinked it is necessary to find the effect of each of these factors on various types of mortality. Cox proportional regression model [13] enables us to find the net effect by adjusting each covariate while controlling for other factors used in the regression. There are different factors that lead to mortality among children at different ages identified by using country level World Fertility Surveys [14]. It is necessary to examine the effects at different ages and also due to different covariates. Hence the regression model is estimated for different age intervals. Often, literature either focuses on neonatal mortality [15-17] or on infant and child mortality [18, 19]. From the conceptual point of view, the proximate and distal determinants at individual, household, community, social and environmental challenges affects the child survival and death. [20].

GENDER AND INTERGENERATIONAL DISPARITIES

Gender bias is one of the crux factors associated with child and infant mortality. A large number of studies suggest that there are gender differentials in child mortality especially in a developing country like India. In the recent census (2011) data we saw a substantial decline in sex ratio. A recent study which uses all rounds of NFHS data showed that factors like feeding, birth order, antenatal care are the critical contributors of gender differentials [21]. Another study found that gender bias is more severe in north western regions and male mortality is higher when the birth order increases [22]. Higher mortality rate was observed for girls in the age group of 2-5 years [23]. The congenital features of child at birth highly influences the first year of childhood, particularly the first month (neonatal period) and recently the prominence is shifted to neonatal mortality (dying within 28 days of birth) which is the most crucial period of child's life. Interestingly, in 2015 almost 45% of world-wide deaths of under-five-year-old occurred during the first month of life [24]. Most (around 99%) of the neonatal deaths occur in low and middle income countries. The major causes of neonatal deaths are infections, birth asphyxia and pregnancy complications of preterm birth and consequently 4 million neonates die every year in low income countries [25].

One of the research papers based on Indian data show that how infant and child mortality is persistent in Indian households using NFHS- 2 data. The death of a sibling in infancy increases the risk of death of the next child in almost 13 States in India even after controlling the effects at family level [26]. Another study with the same data unearthed that short birth intervals between siblings increases the risk of child mortality, and if the eldest sibling is dead, there is a higher amount of risk of dying for the index child. They argue that two children with similar characteristics experience different risk due to the differences in the environmental and accessibility for health care facilities. Among the covariates, they found that interaction variable of maternal education illiterate and short birth interval significantly affects mortality [27]. Similarly, another paper found out that a 10% increase in birth interval will reduce the likelihood of death by 0.45 percentage points [28]. With the same dataset, another study examined the causes of child mortality using Cox hazard regression models where they report that the practice of sex selection prevails in northern states and demographic factors such as residence, region, state have adjusted effects on infant mortality, whereas birth order reflected a U-shaped curve with three and more birth order shows lower mortality [29]. With same methodology, all three rounds of NFHS data are examined for the scheduled tribes in rural areas. Hazard rate was higher for male children and 42% higher when there is an increase in birth order of the child and the literate women were facing 40% less hazard of infant mortality [30].

From the literature it is clear that gender, birth order, birth interval, mother's age, height and weight are prominent factors associated with child mortality. Though some studies have analyzed these factors, none of them have looked into the role of mother's dietary pattern and influence of domestic violence on child mortality. Moreover, the influence of gender and birth order are analyzed separately in previous works which unearth more evidences suggesting that later born children are dying more in India and even if they survive they perform poor in nutrition [31]. It is highly necessary to shed more light that at higher birth order, females have survival advantage than males. This paper tries to address this by combining these two variables and finds striking results which will be discussed in the results section.

SOCIO-ECONOMIC DISPARITIES

All those factors which are not related to birth and genital characteristics such as demographic, socio-economic, health seeking behavior and environmental factors are also found to influence child survival. Children who live in socio-economically deprived community or neighborhood (same environmental conditions) face a higher risk of infections and death [32]. In Ethiopia (second largest populated country in Africa), the risk of neonatal mortality is higher for males and those children who were born in winter season for young age mothers (below 18 years). In rural Ghana, the late initiation of breastfeeding increases the risk of neonatal mortality by 2.4 times [33]. Additionally, most of the literary works assumes even though the child's age is increasing, impacts on mortality over age remain same. There is a strong correlation between demographic and socio-economic characteristics which explained 43.81% of variance through Principal Component Analysis (PCA) in Tanzania for infant and child mortality [34].

Mortality burden was analyzed using the NFHS-2 data where the results highlighted the fact that it is higher in economically disadvantaged and lower income groups. They observed a substantial differential in the mortality rates between the richest and the poorest sections of the society and also found that mortality risks were higher for girls with an odds ratio of 1.33 [23]. The variations in inequality of child mortality burden is explored at the district level with the census data which elucidates the fact that access to hospitals and safe drinking water in highly developed districts increase the inequality in reduction of child mortality. Further, more Muslims were concentrated in developed districts during 1981 and 1991 census and contributed to the reduction in child mortality. On similar lines, the survival advantage of Muslim children was explained by using first two rounds of NFHS data. The genetic built of Muslim women and the non-vegetarian diet and their higher concentration in developed urban areas reduces the mortality risk of their children than their Hindu counterparts [35, 36].

Another dimension for the cause of mortality was analyzed and the paper throws light on the fact that the children of those who experienced domestic violence are at higher risk of death especially in perinatal and neonatal stages. The risk is 68% higher than the women who reported no violence [37]. Among these factors, from the above literature it is evident that there are unresolved puzzles that still remain in terms of religion and open defecation. This paper tries to throw some interesting facts by regenerating these variables at Primary Sampling Unit level.

The past literature either focuses on child or infant mortality. Even in analyzing the causes, the focus is specific to Scheduled Tribes or religion or rural areas [28]. Most of these studies were carried out by using NFHS-2 data. Even though the child poses unique health endowment and resides in the household unit, which in turn is a unit of community, child survival is directly or indirectly influenced by the factors at various levels within the social setup of the community. Therefore, this paper for the first time is making a richer contribution by analyzing the NFHS-3 data by considering all age specific mortality and particularly establishing the relationship between gender and birth order to find out which children survive more.

The recent United Nations report found out that almost 70% of the childhood death occur within the first year of life and in that, 30% of neonatal deaths occur in India. This shows that even after the introduction of successful childhood interventions, we still lack pace in the reduction of mortality. Despite the prominent progress, there is a great deal of stagnation and disparity in reducing mortality rates across the world which necessitates the policies and frameworks at macro level (political) to be linked with micro level (community/household/individual) as there are a lot of variations across States, districts, communities and households. Therefore, this paper makes a contribution by analyzing age specific mortality by allowing the impacts of covariates to change with hazard regression model where time varying covariates can be introduced in the model.

The specific objectives are as follows to,

1. Examine the relative importance of gender differentials effects through birth order rankings on age specific mortality rates.
2. Analyze to what extent the intergenerational transmission factors contribute to age specific mortality rates.
3. Evaluate the effect of domestic violence on age specific mortality rates.

DATA AND METHODOLOGY

National Family Health Survey (NFHS-3) data are used. This dataset is alike the Demographic Health Surveys (DHS) which spreads across almost 80 countries. The entire analysis was child based and restricted to births in the last five years before the survey. The study considered children in the age group of 0-59 months old. Nearly 51,555 live births were recorded since January 2000. Out of the total women 124385 in the age group of 15-49 interviewed, 29.6% of the women reported at least 1 live birth during the interview period.

Survival Analysis

Survival analysis is a statistical method or tool used to analyze time to event data. An event will be the interest of our study. In our study, the event we considered is death of the child; other events may include mileage of cars, infection of disease and its diagnosis, drug treatment etc. that is the time from onset of disease infection to death or time from drug given to death. This analysis is different from other analysis because either the individual or person must wait till the event to occur; where before the time frame of study, some individuals/child will not have faced the event, so the data will always be incomplete. [39] suggest that using other methods of analysis for this incomplete data like ordinary regression models will not yield appropriate results because of the dropout of observations within the study period. This leads to the concept of censoring which is of three types namely right, left and interval censoring.

The Survival Function

Given T, a random variable time, and then the survival function is,

$$S(t) = P(T > t) = 1 - F(t) = 1 - \int_0^t f(u)du \tag{1}$$

Where f(t) and F(t) are the probability density and cumulative density function of a distribution. We are interested in the probability of the child to survive to time t.

The Hazard Function

This helps us to get the child/individual who have not faced death, or those who will be at risk of experiencing death, so the probability of the child will be within the interval [t, t+dt], which is denoted as h (t) dt. So the hazard function will be,

$$h(t) = \lim_{\Delta t \to 0} \left(\frac{1}{\Delta t}\right) P(t \leq T < t + \Delta t | T \geq t) \ldots \quad (2)$$

This shows that if the event does not occur, it will occur within the interval {t, t+dt} which gives the instantaneous occurrence of time. This function will take any non negative shape (increasing, downward, U-shaped) which depends on the survival data. If the function is cumulated over time, then it is known as cumulative hazard function. It is the inverse of the survival function.

$$\lambda(t) = \frac{f(t)}{S(t)}$$

There are various methods involved in the survival analysis. Parametric methods such as exponential distribution, log-normal, log-logistic, Weibull and Gamma distribution are all used to estimate this analysis. Among the regression models, Weibull, Exponential and Cox Proportional models are used to estimate the hazard functions. In this, both Weibull and the Exponential models assume that hazard is constant over time and the duration of time dependency will not be taken into account.

Proportional hazards regression, also called Cox regression, helps us to model the incidence or hazard rate depending on the outcome. In this study, the outcome is death of the child (i.e.,) child mortality. It differs from the logistic regression as it estimates the odds ratio whereas the Cox model estimates the hazard ratio. In this model, hazard ratio is both the function of time as well as the independent variables for example gender, education, residence etc. thereby allowing certain heterogeneity. The major advantage of using this model is that adjusted covariates to risk (hazard) can be estimated. It can be used both for discrete as well as continuous measures and variables which change over time, i.e., time dependent variables can also be introduced into the model. It is an appropriate tool for censoring observations. Another major reason to use this methodology is due to the nesting behavior in the dataset, where child is nested to household, household is nested to community/PSU, PSU is nested to region, and region is nested to a State. All these differences can be captured through this model.

We conceptualize hazard as a continuous function, λ (t) a time-specific hazard rate (failures per person per unit time) for an infinitesimally small time interval centered on time t. Alternatively, at the individual level, λ (t) may be thought of as the probability of failure per unit time.

The general form of the hazard model is

$$\lambda\, x\,(t) = \lambda_0(t)\,.\,C\,x(t)\ldots \tag{3}$$

Where λ_0 (t) denotes a baseline hazard function, which represent the hazard for person for all the explanatory variables as zero. x denotes a set of independent covariates, and $C\,x(t)$ is a multiplier specific to persons with the set x of characteristics. Let $\lambda\,(t\,|X_{1i}, X_{2i}, \ldots, X_{Ki})$ denote the hazard function for the ith child at time t, $i = 1, 2, 3, \ldots, n$, where the K regressors are denoted as $X_{1i}, X_{2i}, \ldots, X_{Ki}$. The baseline hazard function at time t, i.e., when $X_{1i} = 0$, $X_{2i} = 0, \ldots, X_{Ki} = 0$, is denoted as $\lambda_0(t)$. Even though the baseline function is not specified, it must be positive. By dividing both sides with $\lambda_0(t)$ and taking logs, we will get the hazard ratio.

$$\ln\left(\frac{\lambda x(t)}{\lambda_0(t)}\right) = b_1X_1 + b_2X_2 + B_3X_3 + \cdots .\, b_kX_k\ldots \tag{4}$$

The hazard ratio $\left[\frac{\lambda_1(t)}{\lambda_0(t)}\right]$ can be regarded as the relative risk of the event occurring at time t. The ratio of hazard functions can be considered as a ratio of risk functions, so the proportional hazards regression model can be considered as a function of relative risk. Changes in a covariate have multiplicative effect on the baseline risk.

The major assumption of proportional hazards regression is that hazard for any child is a fixed proportion of the hazard for any other child (proportional hazards). If $\lambda_0(t)$ is the hazard function for mortality with all the predictor values equal to zero and $\lambda_1(t)$ is the hazard function for mortality with other values for the predictor variables, then the hazard ratio depends only on the predictor variables and not on time t. This assumption means if a covariate doubles the risk of the event on day one; it also doubles the risk of the event on any other day. The regression equation (4) estimation results are given below.

PRELIMINARY GRAPHS AND TABLES

The Figure 2 line graph depicts the differences in the mortality rates of both neonatal and post neonatal mortality. In Uttar Pradesh, neonatal mortality was 323 per live births whereas it was 204 of post neonatal deaths. Among the North-Eastern States, Assam and Nagaland are performing worse than other States. These differences kindle our interest to find out the causes and necessitate the incorporation of age specific factors into the analysis.

The Figure 3 graph show that there are differences in IMR and U5MR rates; both Uttar Pradesh and Madhya Pradesh had higher rates of infant and under-five-year-old mortality. In Uttar Pradesh itself we lost about 20.8% of children. Even though there is a reduction in 10 years (2005-06 and 2015-16) still India is at lower end in terms of child mortality. Overall, the central and the northern States are worst performers in terms of child survival.

It is inevitable that religion is a part of the socio-economic characteristics and highly influences the mortality rates of children through the behavioral features. This preliminary table gives the life table estimates of children born in Hindus and Muslim categories. In the previous five years of the survey, 35499 children are born Hindus and 8595 children are Muslims. Out of this, 1645 and 349 died respectively within six months. The lost are the children who are not exposed to risk of death within that specified period but anytime they will face the risk. For the lost children, the assumption is that they are exposed for only half of the interval- here it is 3 months instead of 6 months. It is clear from the table that Muslims have a better survival advantage as compared to Hindus. The IMR is the cumulative probability survival that 1-0.9515 equals to 48.5 per 1000 live

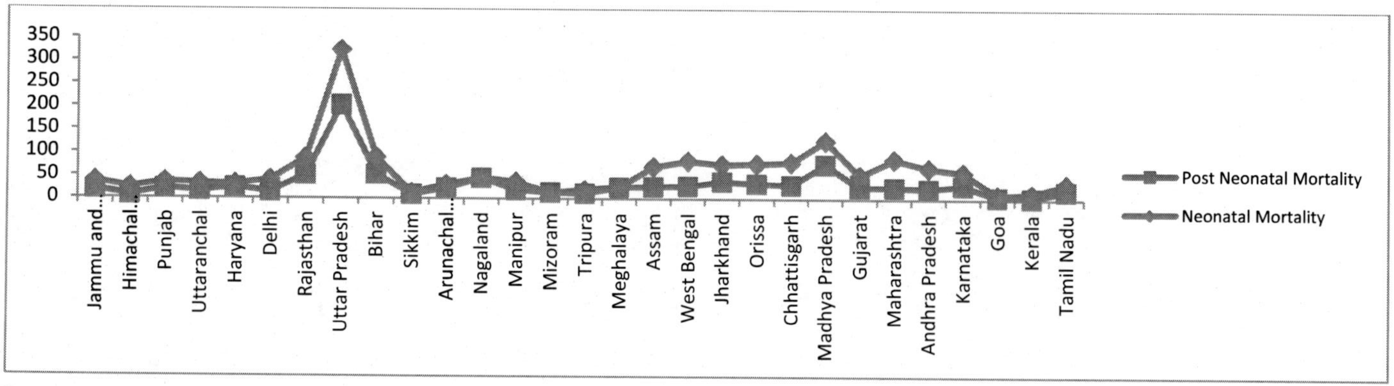

Source: Author's own calculation from NFHS-3.

Figure 2. Neonatal and Post Neonatal mortality per 1000 Live births across States.

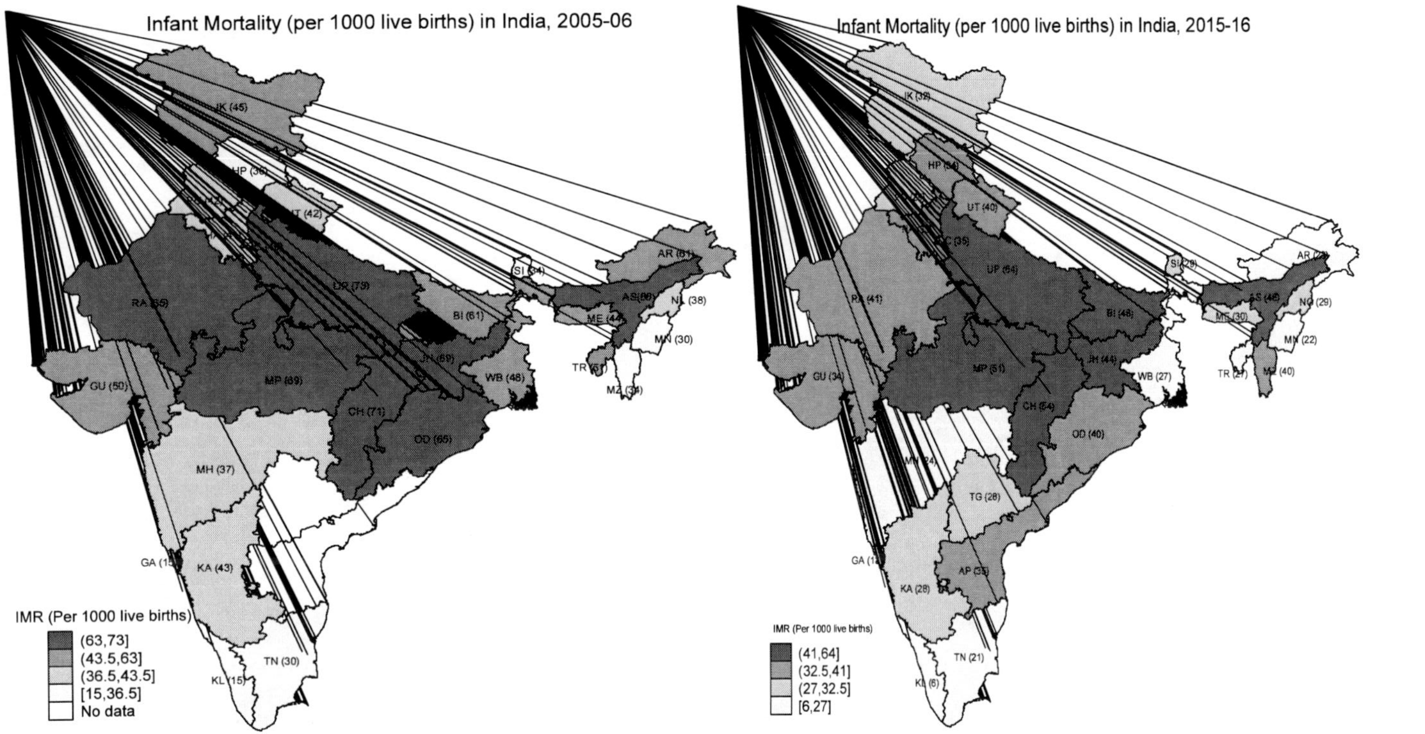

Figure 3. (Continued)

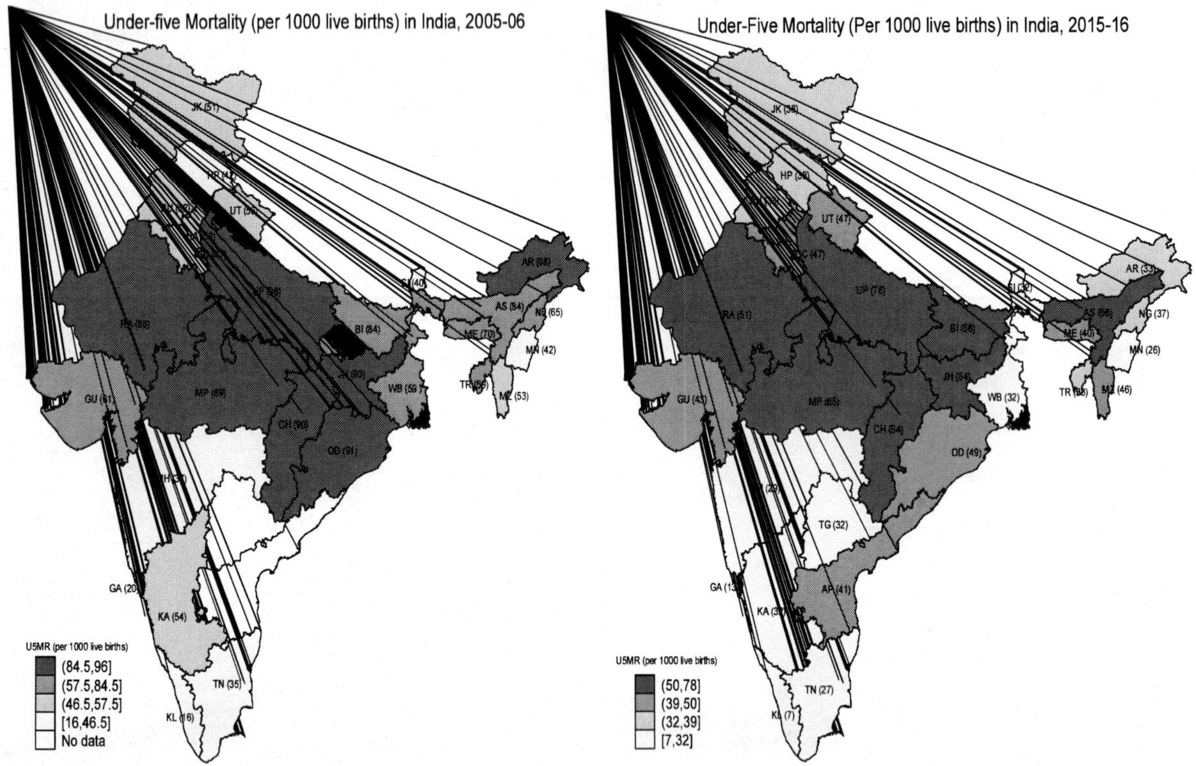

Source: Author's own calculation from NFHS-3 and NFHS-4.

Figure 3. Infant and under-five-year-old mortality per 1000 live births across States.

Table 1. Life table estimates of the children by religion

Interval		Total		Deaths		Lost		Survival	
		Hindus	Muslims	Hindus	Muslims	Hindus	Muslims	Hindus	Muslims
0	5	35499	8595	1645	349	3217	775	0.9515	0.9575
6	11	30637	7471	171	41	3371	797	0.9458	0.9519
12	17	27095	6633	94	25	3257	886	0.9424	0.9481
18	23	23744	5722	39	10	3274	715	0.9407	0.9463
24	29	20431	4997	69	16	3363	839	0.9372	0.943
30	35	16999	4142	1	1	3291	813	0.9372	0.9428
36	41	13707	3328	36	8	3482	864	0.9343	0.9402
42	48	10189	2456	0	0	3354	807	0.9343	0.9402
49	54	6835	1649	8	1	3455	886	0.9329	0.9394
55	59	3372	762	0	0	3372	762	0.9329	0.9394

Source: Author's own calculation from NFHS-3.

births and for Muslims it is 42.5 per 1000 live births at the end of the first year. The under-five-year-old mortality rate (U5MR) will be 1-0.9329 equals to 67.1 per 1000 live births and 60.6 per 1000 live births for Muslims.

STUDY VARIABLES

The NFHS data collects detailed birth history of the individuals where birth year, month, gender, age of the child has been recorded, and whether the child is still alive or dead, if dead, then what age and month the child had died. All these information are used to estimate the survival function. The outcome variable of the study is the risk of death in childhood/infancy which came from the duration of the survival of the child measured in months from birth and analysis is at child-level. Other variables of the study are drawn from the famous work of [20] which is already mentioned in the background section where they categorized the medical determinants as 'proximate' which includes maternal factors, environmental contamination, nutrition deficiency, injury and personal illnesses and the social determinants as 'distal' that includes income, traditions/norms, access to health services and sanitation. Proximate factors such as child sex, birth order, birth size, birth interval, age of mother during child birth and antenatal services are used. Contextual factors of whether child lives in urban/rural areas are also employed and socio-economic factors such as wealth, religion, caste, safe drinking water and sanitation are also included.

The reported birth's in the previous three years before the survey that is from 2000 to 2003 is also included. More specifically, all deaths recorded in 0 to 59 months are considered as failures in the study. The outcome variable is generated with the information on child's 'alive' status and the month at which the child died or till which period the child was alive. Apart from the failures, the children who survived till 28 days (in case of neonatal) or alive after 11 months (Infant mortality) or after 59 months (under-five-year-old) are considered as right-censored for the study.

The main child-mother level variables assessed in this study are sex of the child categorized as male/female, birth order grouped as first birth, second birth and three or more children are interacted with each other to capture who survives more in comparison with the other. Birth interval is dichotomized as less than 24 months or not. Birth size and breastfeeding duration in months are also incorporated. Among mother's characteristics, variables such as mother's education grouped as illiterate, primary, secondary and higher and mother's age at birth are classified as less than 20 years, 20-34 years and greater than or equal to 35 years etc. are included. Other intergenerational characteristics of mother such as her height (in quintiles), BMI, age at first birth, place of delivery, antenatal visits, iron tablets, tetanus injection are all included. Since the data is unavailable on what type of food is consumed by the mother during pregnancy, food habits consumed regularly on normal days are taken as a proxy to measure the diet pattern of the mother and household. And religion and caste variables are also incorporated. Wealth index, a reflector/proxy of a socio-economic status of the household is applied with five quintiles (poorest, poor, middle, richer and richest). Some environment and community level variables such as fuel, sanitation, drinking water are generated at (primary stage units) PSU level which will act as proxy to assess the neighborhood effects. In NFHS, PSU's are the lowest level strata consisting of small administrative units and one PSU might consist of similar characteristics of almost 50 households or units. So the proportion of households of children living in a particular PSU will face particular amount of risk which will be different from other PSU children. Both religion and open defecation variables are converted to PSU levels and interacted with each other to get their net effect. This will help to get a clear assessment of hazard through community level exposures. State dummies are included to control for state fixed effects but the results are not shown here.

REGRESSION RESULTS

The analysis is carried out by following a hierarchical strategy. Initially, individual level proximate factors are introduced into the model and then distal factors and contextual factors are added to retain the significance level of p-value.

Hazard ratios can be interpreted as follows, for dummy variables, the hazard ratio is the ratio of the mortality risk of a child with given characteristics in respect to an infant without those characteristics. For quantitative variables, the hazard ratio is calculated with respect to the baseline hazard function, which is considered as the reference category. The ratio of less than one indicates a reduced risk associated with that factor.

Gender and Intergenerational Differentials

In this study, most of the variables are categorical and the results from Table 2 shows that for the second birth order, males survive better but at higher order of births, females have an advantage of survival than males during their first month of childhood. Strikingly, the results show that among neonatal mortality, girls have 80% chance to survive whereas boys only have 58% at higher order births. But the result is reversed when the duration of survival increases and it is evident that boys have an advantage over girls at higher order births. As discussed in the literature, to some extent the interaction term gives us the clear picture on which child survives more at higher order births at longer duration.

The effect of birth spacing on mortality is one of the most researched area [28, 40, 41] where the results are well- known. Shorter birth intervals will increase the risk of death of the child and it is higher for neonatal deaths and post neonatal deaths (57%). Death clustering in the Indian households is occurring because of shorter birth intervals. Shorter birth intervals also lead to competition in the household resources because there will be children in similar ages and leads to higher risk of infectious diseases.

Another major determinant of survival chance of infancy is the size of child at birth, since 48% of the sample children born in the home that is in a non-institutional setting, birth weight was not assessed properly. It is purely mother's assessment of the child size. Children who are larger and average in size are better off which is shown by the negatively significant coefficient and it is comparatively higher for infant and neonatal mortality.

Regarding mother's characteristics, their place of delivery and age at first birth are one of the prominent factors associated with child mortality. Compared to home delivery, the risk is lower in private hospital and it is very significant for both post neonatal and neonatal mortality. For age of mother at first birth, table 2 shows a mixed pattern where children born to very young mothers and old aged mothers (more than 35 years) are at higher risk whereas the middle aged (24-35) years are producing better offspring and their survival rate is constantly more in all age specific mortality which is indicated by the negatively significant coefficient. The predominant features of intergenerational transmission are mother's height and weight. With the expected sign and hazard, they are highly significant and at higher quintiles, the risk is lower when compared with smaller quintiles. In case of BMI, at higher BMI, the hazard is greater than one reflecting more risk of survival and it is very high (1.44) for neonatal mortality.

Table 2. Regression estimates of Cox regression model

Variables	NNM		PNM		IM		Under-five-year-old	
	Haz. Ratio	Co-eff	Haz. Ratio	Co-eff	Haz. Ratio	Co-eff	Haz. Ratio	Co-eff
*Gender*Birth Order: (1st child Male)*								
Male * 2 child	0.63	-0.463***	0.71	-0.340***	0.76	-0.278***	0.75	-0.277***
Male* More than 3 child	0.56	-0.580***	0.81	-0.210***	0.73	-0.316***	0.74	-0.295***
Female * 1 child	0.7	-0.357***	0.88	-0.128***	0.83	-0.187	0.82	-0.195***
Female* 2 child	0.49	-0.721***	0.13	-0.153***	0.73	-0.313	0.74	-0.296***
Fcmale *More than child	0.45	-0.803***	0.13	-0.237***	0.77	-0.264	0.79	-0.230***
Birth Interval: Less than 24 months(Ref)								
Greater than 24 months	0.57	-0.570***	0.56	-0.574***	0.6	-0.512***	0.6	-0.505***
Birth Size: Smaller than Average(Ref)								
Larger than Average	0.61	-0.122***	0.95	-0.049***	0.88	-0.489***	0.89	-0.142***
Breastfeeding: Never(Ref)								
Less than 3 months	NA	NA	2.58	0.948***	0.5	-0.700***	0.5	-0.687***
3-6 months	NA	NA	1.33	0.289*	0.09	-2.360***	0.1	-2.300***
Greater than 6 months	NA	NA	0.43	-0.853***	0.03	-3.294***	0.05	-2.941***
Place of Delivery: Home(Ref)								
Public Hospital	0.86	-0.146**	0.76	-0.336***	0.93	-0.0657	0.92	-0.82
Private Hospital	0.7	-0.359***	0.71	-0.197**	0.82	-0.007*	0.66	-0.005
Age of Mother at first birth:								
20-34	0.89	-0.118***	0.88	-0.128***	0.87	-0.134***	0.89	-0.122***
More than 35 years	0.42	-0.866***	1.14	0.129***	1.68	.392***	1.67	0.407***
Mother Height: Q1 (Ref)								
Quantile 2	0.86	-0.149***	0.64	-0.450***	0.84	-0.176***	0.85	-0.156***
Quantile 3	0.89	-0.115***	0.59	-0.519***	0.79	-0.240***	0.8	-0.229***

Table 2. (Continued)

Variables	NNM		PNM		IM		Under-five-year-old	
	Haz. Ratio	Co-eff	Haz. Ratio	Co-eff		Haz. Ratio	Co-eff	Haz. Ratio
Quantile 4	0.88	-0.126***	0.72	-0.334***	0.91	-0.097***	0.91	-0.0980***
Quantile 5	0.86	-0.153***	0.61	-0.496***	0.81	-0.213***	0.79	-0.224***
Mother BMI : <18.5(Ref)								
18.5-24.9	0.86	-0.155***	0.86	-0.147***	0.83	-0.187***	0.83	-0.174***
25.0-29.9	1.44	0.361***	1.21	0.193***	1.28	0.246***	1.28	0.254***
Above 30.0	1.32	0.274***	1.43	0.357***	1.27	0.238***	1.23	0.204***
Tetanus Injection: No(Ref)								
Yes	0.62	-0.469***	0.71	-0.337***	0.72	-0.329***	0.72	-0.315***
Iron Tablets: No(Ref)								
Yes	0.83	-0.191***	0.76	-0.273***	0.78	0.253***	0.78	-0.244***
Antenatal Visits	0.7	-0.022***	0.72	-0.021***	0.68	-0.0186***	0.74	-0.018***
Domestic Violence: No(Ref)								
Severe violence	1.04	0.041***	1.31	0.268***	1.11	0.101***	1.08	0.080***
Less Violence	1.08	0.073***	1.13	0.125***	1.03	0.035***	1.06	0.059***
Mother Diet: Low DD(Ref)								
Middle	0.86	-0.156***	0.96	-0.043*	0.93	-0.073	0.94	-0.061
High	0.8	-0.219***	0.9	-0.109	0.91	-0.097***	0.91	-0.098
Mother Education: Illiterate(Ref)								
Primary	0.46	-0.777***	0.44	-0.820***	0.52	-0.663***	0.5	-0.681***
Secondary	0.31	-1.165***	0.27	-1.303***	0.36	-1.018***	0.35	-1.057***
Higher	0.11	-2.186***	0.18	-1.742***	0.18	-1.712***	0.18	-1.726***

Variables	NNM		PNM		IM		Under-five-year-old	
	Haz. Ratio	Co-eff	Haz. Ratio	Co-eff		Haz. Ratio	Co-eff	Haz. Ratio
Father Occupation: Agriculture Workers								
Non-Agri Workers	0.99	-0.006***	1.02	0.0173	0.96	-0.0386	0.95	-0.048***
Wealth: Poorest(Ref)								
Poorer	0.96	-0.394	1.17	0.156	0.95	-0.054	0.95	-0.049
Middle	0.92	-0.088	1.18	0.17	0.96	-0.036	0.96	-0.044
Richer	0.9	-0.101	1.22	0.198	0.95	-0.05	0.93	-0.068
Richest	0.94	-0.06	1.36	0.307	0.98	-0.021	0.96	-0.345
*Open Defecation * Religion: Hindu*OD(Ref)*								
ODMuslim	1.43	0.508***	1.79	0.234	1.78	0.254*	1.75	0.289**
ODChristian	2.56	0.586*	1.97	0.029	1.67	0.405*	2.72	0.334
ODOthers	1.6	0.838**	2.69	0.37	2.63	0.460*	2.64	0.453
Caste: SC(Ref)								
ST	0.89	-0.113	1.11	0.103	1.1	0.099	1.06	0.0927***
OBC	1.01	0.01	0.81	-0.205***	0.99	-0.010*	0.98	-0.017
Others	1.16	0.146*	0.93	-0.073	1.07	0.069	1.05	0.056
PSU Fuel	1.12	0.112***	0.97	-0.033	1.05	0.05	1.03	0.025
PSU water	0.94	-0.064***	0.95	-0.047	1.05	0.05	1.05	0.049
Place of residence: Rural(Ref)								
Urban	0.69	-0.032	0.88	-0.261	0.78	-0.045	0.74	-0.033

Note: *** $p<0.01$, ** $p<0.05$, * $p<0.1$ NA-Not Applicable.

Behavioral Differentials

In the survival analysis, variables like breastfeeding, vaccination, tetanus, antenatal checkups are all predetermined because the decisions are made by mothers only if the child is born. Compared to breast fed children, the non-breast fed infants risk was two-fold high for mortality as well as infectious diseases [42]. It is clear from the table that those children who are breastfed more than 6 months, their risk is lower when compared with other categories. Tetanus is one of the prime reason for neonatal deaths. Infants will get easily infected when unsterilized instruments are used to cut the umbilical cord and there are high chances when the baby is born at unhealthy and unhygienic environments. Every pregnant mother should receive two doses of tetanus injection and the consecutive injection is highly recommended for every three years according to the National Immunization Schedule. From the model, the results show that for those mothers who received tetanus injection, the hazard ratio for their infants are less reflected by negatively significant coefficient. It is highly influencing the neonates with 46% increasing their chances to survive more.

In India, half of the women population is anemic. Especially during pregnancy, it is highly advised to consume iron tablets to gain strength. As expected, the results are favorable for those mothers who had iron tablets. The variable antenatal visits also influences significantly for the mortality risks.

Not much literature documented the role of domestic violence and dietary practices on mortality. These factors are strongly associated with mortality. The behavior of the father like beating, scolding the wife will increase pressure on the mother especially during pregnancy period which leads to complications in birth and the growth of the child. It is obvious from the result that severe violence increases the hazard ratio of the child in survival. The ratios are higher for post neonatal mortality (26.8%) which increases the risk of the child to die. In the modern era, sedentary lifestyle brought changes in the food habits which add more complications in the birth of the child. Compared to lower diversity of food consumption by mother, both middle and high diversity in consumption reduces the mortality risk of the child. It is significant for neonatal mortality (21.9%) and infant mortality (.09%). Education of the mother is the most widely used variable in the literature and the results are not deviating from the past literature as educated mother's infants have lower mortality risk. Since literate mothers are aware of the availability of better health care facilities, nutritious food for healthy child will reduces the risk of dying of the child.

Socio-Economic Differentials

Factors like caste, religion, income are associated with socio-economic differentials on age specific mortality. The wealth quintile variable shows that the richer children are surviving more than their poorest counterparts which is indicated by negative coefficients throughout for all the age specific mortality. However, this variable lost its significance in the full model after the introduction of mother's education and father's occupation in it. Compared to father's who are not in agriculture, the child born in the family whose fathers are professionals are likely to survive more and significant for neonates and infants. But this result show a reversal for post neonatal mortality where the mortality risk is higher for those fathers involved in non-agriculture.

On the longer survival (under-five-year-old and infant), the caste variable shows a mixed pattern when the comparison is with scheduled caste. Scheduled tribe infants are at a higher risk but in neonatal their risk is lower. For OBC and others, neonates are at a higher risk where the hazard ratio is greater than one and they have advantage on longer survival rates.

Environmental Differentials

Other factors like sanitation, safe water, fuel usage, place of residence accounts for the environmental differentials of mortality. The interaction term of open defecation with religion shows an interesting result that compared to Hindu children; all other religions have higher mortality risk from open defecation than Muslim children which explains the answer to the unresolved puzzle that Muslim children have better survival advantage than Hindus. Muslims residing in a better environment and their neighborhood effects will be minimal. More Hindu infants reside in disease and unhealthy environment which leads to mortality. Muslim children also have higher risk from open defecation but comparatively it is lower than other religions. Both the water and the fuel variables are significant for neonatal mortality and show the higher mortality risk on usage of dirty fuel and unsafe drinking water.

CONCLUSION

The study has its own notable strengths that even though the data is ten years old, the implications on the usage of new variables and methods help us to draw specific policy targets for better survival of children. Among the endogenous factors, striking result in this study shows that girls survive more in shorter intervals than boys, but at higher order births, the usual theory of u-shaped curve plays where the later born boys have an advantage to survive. The children who were born at longer birth interval and were larger in size and properly breastfed for the mothers who are educated and middle aged with higher height quintiles and middle range of BMI are having an advantage to survive more. In general, demographic characteristics have substantial effects on mortality up to age five. For the neonatal mortality, the variables such as tetanus injection, mother's high diversity in diet and iron tablets are strongly associated. Hence, as a policy implication to reduce neonatal mortality, focus should be more on the short term policies stressing on the importance of tetanus injection and iron tablets. By concentrating more on family health programs to stress on the longer birth intervals, and stop having children more than four will likely help to increase the survival chances of born children.

For the Under-five-year-old mortality and Infant mortality, the intergenerational variables of mother have high impact, since mother's height and weight reflects both long-term and short-term growth and these variables are strongly associated for longer survival periods. Along with these, the health seeking behavior of antenatal check-ups and institutional delivery helps to curb the U5MR more from the above results. Policy mechanism should be devised to give importance for these infrastructural facilities for reducing U5MR. The strong association of domestic violence on mortality gives us a new connotation to explore more stringent policies in preventing it.

As it is difficult to change the economic pattern and social characteristics in a shorter time [43], policies should focus on more household level programs which target lower economic strata with minimal education [44], support and guidance like sending midwives for treatment of common illness in childhood [45], immunization, home care for the nourishment of babies can be given to reduce mortality. Since malnutrition is the underlying cause of death of many infants where stunting, underweight and wasting paves way for a lot of infections such as diarrhea, fever, cough and other respiratory diseases, strong association is required from social, economical, clinical and environmental, behavioural support to curb the child fatality.

REFERENCES

[1] Rahman, Azizur, and Mahesh Sapkota. Knowledge on vitamin A rich foods among mothers of preschool children in Nepal: impacts on public health and policy concerns. *Science Journal of Public Health* 2, no. 4 (2014): 316-322.

[2] Naline, G., and Brinda Viswanathan. Revisiting the Determinants of Child Anthropometric Indicators in India Using Seemingly Unrelated Regressions Model. *Indian Journal of Human Development* 10, no. 3 (2016): 336-352.

[3] Rahman, Azizur. Rural-urban differentials of childhood malnutrition in Bangladesh. *International Journal of Child Health and Nutrition* (2019): 35-42.

[4] Rahman, Azizur. Geospatial, socioeconomic, demographic and health determinants of childhood mortality in Bangladesh. *Demography India: population - society - economy - environment - interactions,* (2019) 48(2), 74-85.

[5] Rahman, Azizur, Soma Chowdhury, and Delwar Hossain. Acute malnutrition in Bangladeshi children: levels and determinants. *Asia Pacific Journal of Public Health* 21, no. 3 (2009): 294-302.

[6] Megabiaw, Berihun, and Azizur Rahman. Prevalence and determinants of chronic malnutrition among under-5 children in Ethiopia. International Journal of Child Health and Nutrition 2, no. 3 (2013): 230-236.

[7] UNICEF, Levels and Trends in Child Malnutrition: Joint Child Malnutrition Estimates, Key Findings (2019). https://www.who.int/nutgrowthdb/jme-2019-key-findings.pdf.

[8] Roser, Mark. *Child Mortality,* Published online at OurWorldInData.org. Retrieved from: https://ourworldindata.org/child-mortality/ [Online Resource] (2016).

[9] Currie, Janet. Child health in developed countries. *Handbook of health economics* 1 (2000): 1053-1090.

[10] Claeson, Mariam, Eduard R. Bos, Tazim Mawji, and Indra Pathmanathan. Reducing child mortality in India in the new millennium. *Bulletin of the World Health Organization* 78 (2000): 1192-1199.

[11] Bhalotra, Sonia. Links between Childhood Mortality and Economic Growth and Their Implications for Achieving the Millennium Development Goals in India. In *achieving the millennium development goals,* pp. 150-173. Palgrave Macmillan, London, 2008.

[12] Schady, Norbert, and Marc-Francois Smitz. Aggregate economic shocks and infant mortality: New evidence for middle-income countries. *Economics Letters* 108, no. 2 (2010): 145-148.

[13] Cox, David R. Regression models and life-tables. *Journal of the Royal Statistical Society:* Series B (Methodological) 34, no. 2 (1972): 187-202.

[14] Hobcraft, John N., John W. McDonald, and Shea O. Rutstein. Demographic determinants of infant and early child mortality: A comparative analysis. *Population studies* 39, no. 3 (1985): 363-385.

[15] Fikree, Fariyal F., Syed Iqbal Azam, and Heinz W. Berendes. Time to focus child survival programmes on the newborn: assessment of levels and causes of infant mortality in rural Pakistan. *Bulletin of the World Health Organization* 80 (2002): 271-276.

[16] Bhalotra, Sonia R., Christine Valente, and Arthur Van Soest. *Religion and childhood death in India.* CMPO, 2008.

[17] Mekonnen, Yared, Biruk Tensou, Daniel S. Telake, Tedbabe Degefie, and Abeba Bekele. Neonatal mortality in Ethiopia: trends and determinants. *BMC public health* 13, no. 1 (2013): 483.

[18] Bhargava, Alok. Family planning, gender differences and infant mortality: Evidence from Uttar Pradesh, India. *Journal of Econometrics* 112, no. 1 (2003): 225-240.

[19] Maitra, Pushkar. Parental bargaining, health inputs and child mortality in India. *Journal of health economics* 23, no. 2 (2004): 259-291.

[20] Mosley, W. Henry, and Lincoln C. Chen. An analytical framework for the study of child survival in developing countries. *Population and development review* 10, no. 0 (1984): 25-45.

[21] Kuntla, Shrikant, Srinivas Goli, and Kshipra Jain. Explaining sex differentials in child mortality in India: trends and determinants. *International Journal of Population Research* 2014 (2014).

[22] Arokiasamy, Perianayagam. Regional patterns of sex bias and excess female child mortality in India. *Population* 59, no. 6 (2004): 831-863.

[23] Subramanian, S. V., Shailen Nandy, Michelle Irving, Dave Gordon, Helen Lambert, and George Davey Smith. The mortality divide in India: the differential contributions of gender, caste, and standard of

living across the life course. *American Journal of Public Health* 96, no. 5 (2006): 818-825.

[24] World Health Organization. World Health Statistics 2016: Monitoring Health for the Sustainable Development Goals. *World Health Organization* (2016).

[25] Lawn, Joy E., Igor Rudan, and Craig Rubens. Four million newborn deaths: is the global research agenda evidence-based?. *Early human development* 84, no. 12 (2008): 809-814.

[26] Arulampalam, Wiji, and Sonia Bhalotra. Sibling death clustering in India: state dependence versus unobserved heterogeneity. *Journal of the Royal Statistical Society:* Series A (Statistics in Society) 169, no. 4 (2006): 829-848.

[27] Whitworth, Alison, and Rob Stephenson. Birth spacing, sibling rivalry and child mortality in India. *Social science & medicine* 55, no. 12 (2002): 2107-2119.

[28] Bhalotra, Sonia, and Arthur Van Soest. Birth-spacing, fertility and neonatal mortality in India: Dynamics, frailty, and fecundity. *Journal of Econometrics* 143, no. 2 (2008): 274-290.

[29] Pandey, Arvind, Minja Kim Choe, Norman Y. Luther, Damodar Sahu, and Jagdish Chand. *Infant and Child Mortality in India: National Family Health Survey Subject Reports Number 11.* International Institute of Population Sciences: Mumbai (1998).

[30] Sahu, Damodar, Saritha Nair, Lucky Singh, B. K. Gulati, and Arvind Pandey. Levels, trends & predictors of infant & child mortality among Scheduled Tribes in rural India. *The Indian journal of medical research* 141, no. 5 (2015): 709.

[31] Jayachandran, Seema, and Rohini Pande. Why are Indian children so short?. No. w21036. *National Bureau of Economic Research,* 2016.

[32] Aremu, Olatunde, Stephen Lawoko, Tahereh Moradi, and Koustuv Dalal. Socio-economic Determinants in Selecting Childhood Diarrhoea Treatment Options in Sub-Saharan Africa: A Multilevel Model. *Italian Journal of Pediatrics* 37, no. 1 (2011): 13.

[33] Edmond, Karen M., Charles Zandoh, Maria A. Quigley, Seeba Amenga-Etego, Seth Owusu-Agyei, and Betty R. Kirkwood.

Delayed breastfeeding initiation increases risk of neonatal mortality. *Pediatrics* 117, no. 3 (2006): e380-e386.

[34] Adam, Hans and Akarro, Rocky, RJ Assessment of Demographic and Socio Economic Factors on Infant and Child Mortality in Tanzania, *The International Journal's Research Journal of Social Science and Management,* (2013),2(11).

[35] Bhalotra, Sonia, Christine Valente, and Arthur Van Soest. The puzzle of Muslim advantage in child survival in India. *Journal of Health Economics* 29, no. 2 (2010): 191-204.

[36] Brainerd, Elizabeth, and Nidhiya Menon. Religion and health in early childhood: Evidence from South Asia. *Population and Development Review* 41, no. 3 (2015): 439-463.

[37] Koenig, Michael A., Rob Stephenson, Rajib Acharya, Lindsay Barrick, Saifuddin Ahmed, and Michelle Hindin. Domestic violence and early childhood mortality in rural India: evidence from prospective data. *International journal of epidemiology* 39, no. 3 (2010): 825-833.

[38] Van der Klaauw, Bas, and Limin Wang. Child mortality in rural India. *World Bank Policy Research Working Paper* 3281 (2004).

[39] Aalen, Odd, Ornulf Borgan, and Hakon Gjessing. *Survival and Event History Analysis: A Process Point of View.* Springer Science & Business Media, 2008.

[40] DaVanzo, Julie, Abdur Razzaque, Mizanur Rahman, Lauren Hale, Kapil Ahmed, Mehrab Ali Khan, Golam Mustafa, and Kaniz Gausia. The effects of birth spacing on infant and child mortality, pregnancy outcomes, and maternal morbidity and mortality in Matlab, Bangladesh. *Technical Consultation and Review of the Scientific Evidence for Birth Spacing* (2004).

[41] Kozuki, Naoko, and Neff Walker. Exploring the association between short/long preceding birth intervals and child mortality: using reference birth interval children of the same mother as comparison. *BMC public health* 13, no. S3 (2013)

[42] Sankar, Mari Jeeva, Bireshwar Sinha, Ranadip Chowdhury, Nita Bhandari, Sunita Taneja, Jose Martines, and Rajiv Bahl. Optimal

breastfeeding practices and infant and child mortality: A systematic review and meta-analysis. *Acta paediatrica* 104 (2015): 3-13.

[43] Rahman, Azizur. Estimating small area health-related characteristics of populations: A methodological review. *Geospatial Health*, *12*(2017): 3-14. [495]. https://doi.org/10.4081/gh.2017.495

[44] Das, Sumonkanti., Azizur Rahman, Ashraf Ahamed, and S. T. Rahman. Multi-level models can benefit from minimizing higher-order variations: An illustration using child malnutrition data. *Journal of Statistical Computation and Simulation*, *89*(2019): 1090-1110. https://doi.org/10.1080/00949655.2018.1553242

[45] Rahman, Azizur. Significant risk factors for childhood malnutrition: Evidence from an Asian developing country. *Science Journal of Public Health*, *4*(2016): 16-27.

In: Malnutrition
Editor: Azizur Rahman
ISBN: 978-1-53617-597-4

Chapter 6

CHILDHOOD UNDERWEIGHT IN RURAL BANGLADESH

Ashfikur Rahman[1,*] and Sazedur Rahman[2], MD
[1]Development Studies Discipline, Khulna University, Khulna, Bangladesh
[2]Statistics Discipline, Khulna University, Khulna, Bangladesh

ABSTRACT

Weight-for-age or underweight is a chief cause of global disease burden among children aged under five years. It is associated with child mortality and morbidity and it obstructs the child's growth and blockage the way of cognitive development which thus the result of chronic diseases in later life. In Bangladesh, underweight is a major public health problem and it is one of the highest prevalent countries in the world. However, children in rural communities in Bangladesh are more prone to be underweight compared to the children of urban areas. Therefore, this study was an endeavor to examine the factors associated with underweight in rural Bangladeshi children. Nationally representative data from the Bangladesh Demographic and Health Survey (BDHS) 2014 data

* Corresponding Author's Email: ashfikurr@gmail.com.

set was used for the study. A total of 4881 under-five year's aged children from rural areas were included in this study. An estimated 35.1% of children aged under five years were underweight, whereas 26.1% moderately and 9% were severely underweight. Chi-square test was performed to examine the association between weight-for-age status and the selected covariates. Multinomial logistic regression was used to identify the associated factors with childhood underweight. Geographic division, child age, size at birth, fever and diarrhea episode, mother's age at first birth, maternal BMI (kg/m2), father's education, wealth index, toilet facilities and the number of under-5 children were significantly associated with different form of underweight. As malnutrition is an amendable disease, therefore, it is important and implements with enough interventions to prevent, diagnose and treat malnutrition. To sum up, it worth pointing out that health policymakers should put emphasis on the national perspective while designing the health policies and programs for children in rural Bangladesh.

Keywords: underweight, weight-for-age, under-5, risk factors, Bangladesh

INTRODUCTION

Childhood malnutrition or undernutrition measured as poor anthropometric status is internationally documented as a vital public health indicator for monitoring nutritional status and health of the populations which is directly linked with the economic empowerment of a country. There is strong empirical evidence that malnutrition is significantly associated with delayed mental development and retardation [1-5], and several studies have shown an affiliation between poor nutritional status and poor academic performance as well as concentrated intellectual attainment [6-11].

Three anthropometric parameters are widely used to measure the nutritional status of the children: height for age (stunting), weight for height (wasting) and weight for age (underweight). Underweight, defined based on weight-for-age, is a composite measure of stunting and wasting and is recognized as the indicator for assessing changes in the magnitude of malnutrition over time [12]. Under-five (U5) aged is the most susceptible age for children to be affected by undernutrition, and nutritional status during early childhood is sensitively used to determine the whole public health status of a country. Since weight-for-age is a composite index of weight-for-height and height-for-age, it does not distinguish between acute malnutrition (wasting) and chronic malnutrition (stunting). A child can be underweighted for his or her earlier age because the child is stunted, is wasted, or both. Therefore, weight-for-age is an overall indicator of a population's nutritional health.

Underweight is considered a significant culprit of causing child death globally. Black et al. 2013 documented that only underweight accounts for 14% of total child death [12] globally. In 1990 worldwide, almost 159 million U5 children were underweighted while with a 36% decreasing rate, the number was 100 million in 2011 [13]. In 2011, the average rate of underweight among children aged under five years was 16%, but it remained high in south-central Asia (30%) [14]. Based on literature three south Asian countries India, Pakistan and Bangladesh are in the peak position of underweight conditions.

Identifying the significant determinants of underweight has been of interest to researchers over a long time. To be underweight there have multidimensional causes and most of them are interrelated, but they may be often differed due to countries' socioeconomic and geographical circumstances, consequently, local research highlighting on examining the root causes of childhood underweight is recommended. However following the factors are commonly found and documented in public health literature, maternal education [13-18], paternal education [10-11, 17-19], low maternal body mass index [15-21], father's occupation [16-19], age of child [9, 12-13, 15 21-23], sex of the child [14], multiple births [17], small size at birth [12-13, 19, 23], birth interval [13, 16, 23], birth order [14-15, 21], child feeding index [9, 12, 24], incidence of fever [9], respiratory illness [9, 15], diarrhea [9, 12], mother exposure to mass media [13, 15], antenatal care visit [11], number of under-five children [15], toilet facility [15], household wealth status [6, 9-10, 14-16, 25] and region of residence [11, 13, 15, 23].

In the past few decades Bangladesh has done well in improving socio-economic status but still, a large number of populations are living below the poverty threshold and it is known by all poverty leads to poor-socio-economic status. And poor socioeconomic status like poverty is significantly associated with childhood underweight [20]. It can be called a vicious cycle of childhood poor nutritional status. Though the rate of childhood malnutrition has been found decreasing in recent years the situation is still worse than any other developing country around the world. The data of 2014 BDHS pointed out that the prevalence rate of underweight was 33% in 2014 and in 2011 it was 41% [20] which is higher than any other developing country [26]. This extent of underweight is above the threshold 'very high' [10]. The children in rural communities in Bangladesh are more vulnerable to be underweight than urban children [27]. The prevalence of underweight was higher among rural children 35% than that of the urban children 28% [20%]. Indeed, a number of studies done in Bangladesh, reported that household socioeconomic status, mother's biological characteristics, infant feeding practice were associated with underweight.

Keeping knowledge about the updated determinants of underweight is supremely needed for the better pregnancy outcome and improving child survival capability of Bangladeshi children. The prime uniqueness of this such study is that the findings are very new because a similar study had not found elsewhere which had directly worked with rural people. In addition, it covers a wide range of nationally representative data thus it is possible to generalize the findings, that would be conducive to know about the public health situation of the country like Bangladesh. Therefore, we designed this present study is an endeavor to ascertain the most associated factors that contribute to underweight in rural Bangladeshi children to help policymakers to reduce the overall burden of malnutrition.

METHODS

This study performed a secondary data analysis collected in 2014 by NIPORT across the country [26] with a cross-sectional method. The survey was the seventh national-level demographic and health survey and conducted by the National Institute of Population Research and Training (NIPORT) of the Ministry of Health and Family Welfare of Bangladesh and one of the specific objectives of this survey was to provide updated and reliable estimates of the nutritional status of under-5 children. Two-stage stratified sampling method was used in both rural and urban areas the expected number of households was 18000. A total of 17863 ever-married women aged 15-49 were interviewed with a response rate of 98 percent. A sum up 7886 under-5 children's information was available where 5398 (68.45%) were rural children. Among these children, 517 subjects were excluded due to huge missing cases and finally, 4881 child-pairs information was included for the study purpose.

Based on the World health standard growth, the underweight children were identified by the anthropometric measurement weight-for-age (underweight) on the basis of Z-score of weight-for-age (WAZ) then categorized into nourished, moderately underweight, and severely underweight if his/her Z-score for WAZ was respectively exposed in the ranges: Z-score ≥ -2.0, $-3.0 \leq$ Z-score < -2.0 and Z-score < -3.0. From the height, weight, and age of the children, the Z-scores were calculated using the WHO AnthroPlus Software (version 3.2.2, 2011).

A set of demographic and socioeconomic and biological factors were considered in this study: division, sex of child, child age, size at birth, fever, maternal age at first birth, maternal BMI, maternal education, paternal education, maternal occupation, paternal occupation, wealth index, mother exposure to TV, toilet facilities, number of under-5 children, and birth order. The association test was performed using Pearson's chi-square test. Then we used multinomial logistic regression models to estimate the relative risk ratio (RRR) for any underweight conditions. The level of significance was set at $p<0.05$. Data were analyzed using STATA version 12.

PREVALENCE OF CHILDHOOD UNDERWEIGHT IN RURAL BANGLADESH

According to the report of BDHS 2014, 35.1% of under-5 children in rural Bangladesh were underweight, where 26.1% were moderately underweight and 9% were severely underweight. Table1 reveals the prevalence of moderate and severe underweight according to the selected covariates. The prevalence of moderate underweight was highest in the Barisal division (27.92%) and severe underweight was highest in the Sylhet division (13.1%). Twenty percent of children under age 12 months were underweight and the rate of underweight continues to increase with age, peaking at 40% at age 35-59 months. The data shows a strong association between underweight and their perceived birth size. The prevalence of both the moderate and severe underweight was higher among children perceived by their mothers as smaller than the average size at birth compared to the children perceived by their mothers more than the average size at birth. The prevalence of overall underweight was higher among the children who were suffered from recent fever. The percentage of children with moderate and severe underweight increases with decreasing maternal BMI levels, maternal education, paternal education, household wealth index, mother's exposure to television and toilet facilities. For example, compared to the children whose mother's BMI was equal or greater than 18.50 kg/m2, the prevalence of both the moderate (32% *vs.*24%) and severe underweight (14.6% *vs.* 7%) was higher in the children whose mother's BMI were less than 18.50 kg/m2. The percentage of both the moderate (31.2%) and severe underweight (13.7%) was the highest among uneducated mothers. The prevalence rate of both moderate and severe underweight was the highest (30.5% and 10.5%) among children whose mothers were involved in working agricultural works. Further, the frequency of both moderate and severe underweight was the highest (29.4% and 12%) among children whose birth order was 4rth or above the percentage of severe underweight was lower (8.3%) in the household with having had only one under-5 child.

Table 1. Background characteristics of the children and the prevalence of underweight (n=4881)

Characteristics	Overall N (%)	Underweight		Nourished N (%)	*p*-value[1]
		Moderate, N (%)	Severe, N (%)		
Division					0.000
Barisal	591(12.11)	165(27.92)	51(8.63)	375(63.45)	
Chittagong	912(18.68)	247(27.08)	87(9.54)	578(63.38)	
Rajshahi	617(12.64)	162(26.26)	48(7.78)	407(65.96)	
Rangpur	657(13.46)	182(27.70)	58(8.83)	417(63.45)	
Sylhet	842(17.25)	235(27.90)	110(13.1)	497(59.0)	
Khulna	521(10.67)	112(21.50)	32(6.14)	377(72.36)	
Dhaka	741(15.18)	172(23.21)	54(7.29)	515(69.5)	
Sex of child					0.731
Male	2501(51.24)	642(25.67)	224(8.96)	1635(65.37)	
Female	2380(48.76)	633(26.6)	216(9.08)	1531(64.33)	
Child age (months)					0.000
0-11	951(19.48)	155(16.3)	46(4.84)	750(78.86)	
12-21	874(17.91)	211(24.1)	90(10.3)	573(65.56)	
22-34	1042(21.35)	296(28.41)	105(10.08)	641(61.52)	
35-59	2014(41.26)	613(30.44)	199(9.88)	1202(59.68)	
Size at birth					0.000
<Average	582(11.92)	181(31.1)	99(17.01)	302(51.89)	
≥Average	4299(88.08)	1094(25.45)	341(7.93)	2864(66.62)	
Fever					0.000
No	3047(62.43)	777(25.5)	235(7.71)	2035(66.79)	
Yes	1834(37.57)	498(27.15)	205(11.18)	1131(61.67)	
Maternal age (years) at first birth					0.000
<20	3712(76.05)	999(26.91)	364(9.81)	2349(63.28)	
≥20	1169(24.95)	276(23.61)	76(6.5)	817(69.89)	
Maternal BMI ((kg/m^2)					0.000
≤ 18.50	1240(25.4)	400(32.26)	182(14.68)	658(53.06)	
>18.50	3641(74.6)	875(24.03)	258(7.09)	2508(68.86)	
Maternal education					0.007
No education	818(16.76)	255(31.17)	112(13.69)	451(55.13)	
Primary	1461(29.93)	448(30.66)	153(10.47)	860(58.86)	
Secondary	2252(46.14)	508(22.56)	162(7.19)	1582(70.25)	
Higher	350(7.17)	64(18.29)	13(3.71)	273(78.0)	
Paternal education					0.000
No education	1355(27.76)	415(30.63)	197(14.54)	743(54.83)	
Primary	1590(32.58)	452(29.43)	141(8.87)	997(62.7)	
Secondary	1431(29.3)	303(21.19)	83(5.8)	1045(73.01)	
Higher	505(10.35)	105(20.79)	19(3.76)	381(75.45)	

Table 2. (Continued)

Characteristics	Overall N (%)	Underweight		Nourished N (%)	*p*-value[1]
		Moderate, N (%)	Severe, N (%)		
Maternal occupation					0.016
Household	3554(72.81)	895(25.18)	318(8.95)	2341(65.87)	
Agricultural Sector	770(15.78)	235(30.52)	81(10.52)	454(58.96)	
Non-agricultural Sector	427(8.75)	113(26.46)	31(7.26)	283(66.28)	
Service Sector	130(2.66)	32(24.62)	10(7.69)	88(67.69)	
Paternal occupation					0.017
Agriculture sector	1574(32.25)	458(29.1)	176(11.18)	940(59.72)	
Non-agricultural sector	978(20.04)	256(26.18)	120(12.27)	602(61.55)	
Business	1146(23.48)	284(24.78)	74(6.46)	788(68.76)	
Service sector	1183(24.24)	277(23.42)	70(5.92)	836(70.67)	
Wealth index					0.000
Poor	2530(51.83)	776(30.67)	310(12.25)	1444(57.08)	
Middle	1094(22.41)	279(25.5)	80(7.31)	735(67.18)	
Rich	1257(25.75)	220(17.5)	50(3.98)	987(78.52)	
Mother exposure to TV					0.000
No	3496(71.62)	992(28.38)	368(10.53)	2136(61.10)	
Yes	1385(28.38)	283(20.43)	72(5.2)	1030(32.53)	
Toilet facilities					0.000
No facilities	162(3.32)	57(35.19)	28(17.28)	77(47.53)	
Hanging toilet	197(4.04)	69(35.03)	32(16.24)	96(48.73)	
Pit toilet	4173(85.49)	1096(26.26)	365(8.75)	2712(64.99)	
Flush toilet	349(7.15)	53(15.19)	15(4.3)	281(80.52)	
Number of under-5 children					0.003
1	3221(65.99)	835(25.92)	268(8.32)	2118(65.76)	
2	1364(27.95)	378(27.71)	131(9.6)	855(62.68)	
≥ 3	296(6.06)	62(20.95)	41(13.85)	193(65.2)	
Birth order					0.000
1st	1788(36.63)	442(24.72)	141(7.89)	1205(67.39)	
2nd	1426(29.22)	377(26.44)	112(7.85)	937(65.71)	
3rd	806(16.51)	203(25.19)	84(10.42)	519(64.39)	
≥ 4th	861(17.64)	253(29.38)	103(11.96)	505(58.65)	

[1]*p*-value is obtained from chi-square test.

RISK FACTORS OF CHILDHOOD UNDERWEIGHT IN RURAL BANGLADESH

Multinomial logistic regression was used to reveal the risk factors for moderate and severe underweight where the nourished children were reference category. The results of the logistic regression are placed in Table 2. Results depict that compared with children of the Dhaka division, the children of Chittagong division were 1.37 and 1.54 times more likely to be being moderate underweight and severe underweight respectively. Also, the children of the Sylhet division had a higher risk of being severely underweight in response to children of Dhaka division. Children of a younger age than 35 months were less likely to be moderately and severely underweight than the children of older age (35-59 months). For example, the children of 0-11 months of age were 65% and 78% less likely to be moderately and severely underweight than the children of 35-months of age. The children with less than the average size at birth ran 1.97 times and 3.38 times high risk of being moderately underweight and severely underweight than the children with average or higher than the average size at birth. Children whose fathers had no education were more likely of being severely underweight than those of the children whose fathers had a higher level of education. Further, the children of the mothers had a BMI of less than 18.50 kg/m2 ran 1.58 times and 2.08 times more risk to be moderately and severely underweight children than the mothers having had a BMI 18.50 kg/m2 or above.

The model also found that children who came from poor and middle wealth index household the odds of being underweight were higher compared with children from the richest wealth index. Children belonging to poor indexed households were 2.12 times and in middle indexed household 1.60 times more likely to be severely underweight. Also, the risk of moderate underweight was higher in households without a toilet or with a hanging toilet compared with the household having a flush toilet. Besides, free from recent febrile illness and household having only one under-5 child were protective factors for severe underweight. Furthermore, maternal age at first birth (<20 years) were a significant risk factor for severe underweight in under-5 children.

Table 3. Multinomial logistic regression analysis for moderate and severe underweight

Characteristics	Moderate Underweight		Severe Underweight	
	RRR [95% CI for RRR]	***p*-value**	**RRR [95% CI for RRR]**	***p*-value**
Division				
Barisal	1.20[0.92-1.57]	0.171	1.18[0.76-1.81]	0.454
Chittagong	1.37[1.08-1.74]	0.010	1.54[1.05-2.26]	0.025
Rajshahi	1.05[0.80-1.36]	0.707	0.96[0.62-1.48]	0.864
Rangpur	1.16[0.90-1.51]	0.253	1.08[0.71-1.65]	0.702
Sylhet	1.23[0.95-1.57]	0.103	1.56[1.07-2.27]	0.020
Khulna	0.91[0.68-1.21]	0.530	0.89[0.55-1.44]	0.644
Dhaka (ref.)				
Child age (months)				
0-11	0.35[0.27-0.45]	0.000	0.22[0.14-0.33]	0.000
12-21	0.63[0.51-0.77]	0.000	0.68[0.51-0.92]	0.014
22-34	0.80[0.67-0.96]	0.020	0.74[0.55-0.98]	0.041
35-59 (ref.)				
Size at birth				
<Average	1.97[1.58-2.45]	0.000	3.38[2.51-4.55]	0.000
≥Average (ref.)				
Fever				
No	0.87[0.75-1.00]	0.059	0.65[0.53-0.81]	0.000
Yes (ref.)				
Maternal age (years) at first birth				
<20	1.12[0.95-1.33]	0.160	1.36[1.03-1.80]	0.030
≥20 (ref.)				
Maternal BMI (kg/m^2)				
< 18.50	1.58[1.35-1.84]	0.000	2.08[1.66-2.61]	0.000
≥18.50 (ref.)				
Maternal education				
No education	1.23[0.82-1.84]	0.305	0.99[0.48-2.03]	0.976
Primary	1.30[0.90-1.88]	0.165	0.96[0.48-1.92]	0.919
Secondary	1.02[0.73-1.43]	0.910	0.98[0.51-1.88]	0.962
Higher (ref.)				
Paternal education				
No education	1.02[0.74-1.40]	0.902	1.83[1.01-3.30]	0.044
Primary	0.96[0.72-1.30]	0.836	1.25[0.71-2.22]	0.428
Secondary	0.81[0.61-1.08]	0.158	1.02[0.58-1.80]	0.937
Higher education (ref.)				

Characteristics	Moderate Underweight		Severe Underweight	
	RRR [95% CI for RRR]	***p*-value**	**RRR [95% CI for RRR]**	***p*-value**
Maternal occupation				
Household	0.94[0.61-1.47]	0.819	1.11[0.54-2.28]	0.769
Agricultural Sector	1.12[0.70-1.78]	0.630	1.28[0.60-2.71]	0.521
Non-agricultural Sector	0.95[0.58-1.55]	0.852	0.91[0.41-2.05]	0.836
Service Sector (ref.)				
Paternal occupation				
Agriculture sector	1.11[0.91-1.35]	0.300	1.36[0.99-1.89]	0.058
Non-agricultural sector	0.95[0.76-1.18]	0.668	1.42[1.01-2.00]	0. 053
Business	1.07[0.87-1.30]	0.503	1.00[0.70-1.43]	0.980
Service sector (ref.)				
Wealth index				
Poor	1.66[1.29-2.13]	0.000	2.12[1.38-3.26]	0.001
Middle	1.45[1.15-1.81]	0.001	1.60[1.05-2.40]	0.026
Rich (ref.)				
Mother exposure to TV				
No	1.06[0.81-1.38]	0.579	1.12[0.80-1.56]	0.500
Yes (ref.)				
Toilet facilities				
No facilities	1.76[1.07-2.90]	0.025	1.84[0.86-3.94]	0.113
Hanging toilet	1.68[1.05-2.67]	0.030	1.60[0.77-3.33]	0.207
Pit toilet	1.35[0.97-1.88]	0.076	1.19[0.66-2.14]	0.551
Flush toilet (ref.)				
Number of under-5 children				
1	1.18[0.86-1.62]	0.311	0.62[0.41-0.92]	0.019
2	1.35[0.98-1.86]	0.072	0.75[0.50-1.13]	0.173
≥ 3				
Birth order				
1st	1.06[0.85-1.31]	0.599	1.00[0.72-1.38]	0.999
2nd	1.15[0.92-1.42]	0.212	1.01[0.73-1.41]	0.920
3rd	0.97[0.77-1.23]	0.839	1.12[0.80-1.58]	0.498
≥ 4th (ref.)				

Reference Category: Nourished; ref: Reference; RRR: Relative risk ratios; CI: Confidence interval.

FACTORS ASSOCIATED WITH UNDERWEIGHT

In this study, except for the sex of the children, all the selected covariates were significantly associated with underweight in rural children.

In the multivariate analysis, covariates with a significant association with increased risk for moderate underweight were: geographic division, size at birth, age of the child, maternal BMI, wealth index, household toilet facilities whereas geographic division, size at birth, age of the child, maternal age at first birth, maternal BMI, wealth index, number of under-5 children and recent fever were significantly correlated with severe underweight. Figure 1 shows the associated risk factors for underweight in rural Bangladeshi children.

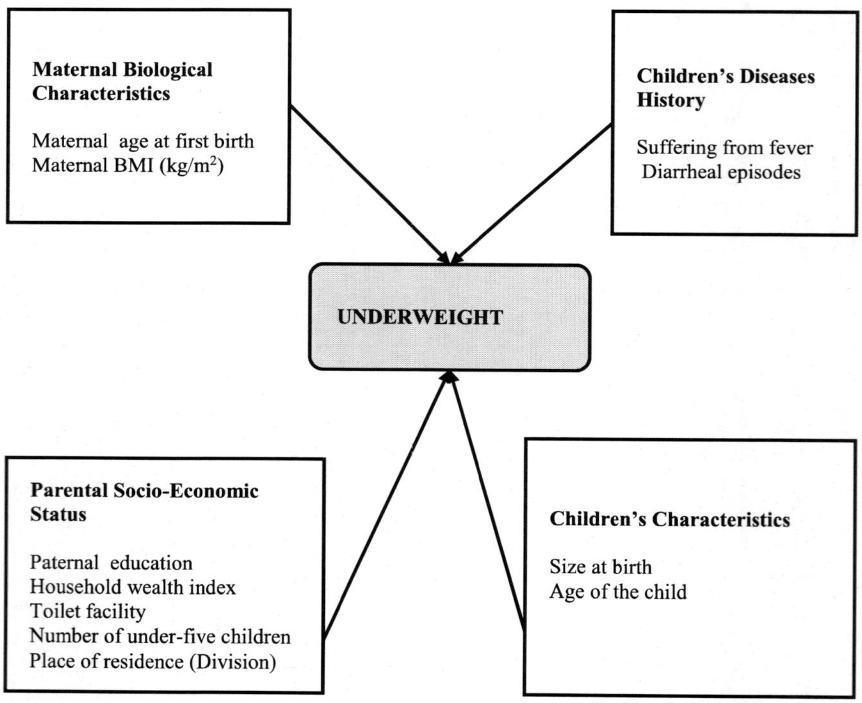

Figure 1. Risk factors for underweight in rural Bangladeshi children.

Division

The current study has established an influential relation between division as geographical location and children to be underweight. The study had found that children of Chittagong were more prone to be underweight in both two forms severe and moderate underweight, whilst, children of Sylhet were more likely to be moderate underweight. Previous studies in Bangladesh also found the place of the region was a significant factor for the cause of childhood underweight [11, 13, 15, 17]. These findings indicate that regional variation in underweight among under-5 children has lasted for a long time in the country. Regional differences in access to medical facilities and proper education, awareness about health and nutrition and socio-demographic status might be the possible reason for this. Therefore, the study recommends that with special plans and policies regional inequalities should be removed throughout the country.

Child Age

The age of the children was found to be an important risk factor for children to be being underweight. Study shows that children's risk of being underweight increased with age, and the highest between the ages of 35–59 months. This finding is supported by a previously done study where the risk of being underweight and severely underweight as highest in the older age children [9, 18, 21-23]. There would have been many reasons behind this relationship between older age and underweight, the possible explanations may be with increasing children's age they start to intake supplementary food along with breast milk. If the complementary food is to be adulterated that can spread various diseases in a child's body which later turns children towards the risk of being underweight [28]. One the other hand, younger aged children are still being breastfed, thereby gaining essential nutrition that renders them less vulnerable to malnourished.

Size at Birth

Mother's perceived child size at birth intrinsically linked with the nutritional status of the child [21], as low birth weight is considered to be an indicator of restricted intrauterine growth and weight [29]. The present study found that children born with smaller than average size at birth ran a higher risk of being underweight compared to those born with larger than the average size at birth. Findings are in line with the previous studies in Bangladesh [13, 21], Nepal [19] and Ghana [18]. Since maternal lack of nutrition is a significant predictor for underweight, effective steps are needed to be taken for improving the maternal nutritional capacity, special attention should be given for rural mothers. Additionally, community health care centers should be modernized with adequate facilities so that they can provide proper services to the rural mothers during the pregnancy period and any forms of emergency as well.

Fever

Children who did not encounter recent fever had less chance of being underweight than those who were suffered from febrile illness. Das and Rahman (2011) also found a significant association between fever and underweight in childhood [15]. This might be children with febrile illnesses are responsible to reduce food intake and loss of fluids which affect the weight of the children [30-31].

Mother's Age (Years) at First Birth

The possibility of underweight was less among children whose mothers were over 20 years compared with those below. The finding is reliable with another study conducted in rural areas in China [32]. This might be since young women are, by and large, less experienced in caregiving and provide unqualified items [32]. Besides, an adolescent mother needs an extra amount of food and nutrients for their growth and development. Consequently, pregnancy during adolescence age may slow down the mother's growth result in an underweight baby [33].

Maternal BMI (kg/m^2)

The risk of underweight was higher among those children whose mothers have had low BMI (<18.5 kg/m2) comparing to BMI ≥18.5 kg/m2. Because maternal BMI has been used as a significant indicator to evaluate the intergenerational health links between a mother and her children. This finding is similar and supports the previous findings that mothers' low BMI affected children's to be underweight [15-21]. As mother's nutritional and health status play a pivotal role in early childhood growth and development [34] and the rural mothers are not so aware of their nutritional status, mother's nutritional status, especially in rural Bangladesh, must be considered during designing any programs or policies regarding improving childhood malnutrition.

Paternal Education

Paternal education had found as a significant predictor of severe underweight. The result is endorsed by other studies and exposed that a lower level of paternal education is closely associated with increasing the odds of child underweight [15-16, 18, 22-28]. Generally, education level is considered as the precondition for household income, because education and to get a better job are related which is the proxy of earning enough income [35] which thus confirm adequate food supply for the family members. In Bangladesh, most of the households are dominated by male-headed and fathers are sometimes the only earning members so it may create an inadequate supply of nutritional foods during pregnancy. Even it may reduce the chance of ANC or PNC. Therefore, dynamic strategies are required to improve father's education that would be conducive to reduce the burden of childhood malnutrition.

Wealth Index

Children come off and living in a higher wealth indexed family had a lower risk of being underweight whereas children of a poor wealth index family had a greater chance of being underweight is inconsistent with previously done studies [6, 16-17, 19-21, 24]. The elucidation could be due to those children in higher wealth index families were more likely to enjoy a better life with adequate foods, medical facilities, and basic amenities. Other reasons might be that high wealth indexed families belong to well-educated father-mother and family members that leads to a greater chance of having basic amenities. Even educated family members are more aware of their upcoming baby and mother's health so this helps the babies to encounter malnourished.

Toilet Facilities

Researchers also observed that the sanitary facility affects childhood malnutrition [12, 20]. An improved well-equipped sanitary facility can develop childhood nutritional status. The results of this study indicate that children in households with poor toilet facilities are more prone to be underweight compared with children from a household with improved toilets. With the agreement of a study in Bangladesh, the findings manifest higher sustainable access to sanitation leads to lower risk for underweight [19]. Access to improved toilets is argued to reduce childhood malnutrition in rural Bangladesh.

Number of Under-5 Children

This study reveals that households with only one under-5 children had about 40% lower risk of severely underweight children than a household with three or more children. The previous study in Bangladesh also showed families with fewer children had a lower proportion of severely underweight children than families with more children [20]. This possible elucidation is to be fewer children means, families can provide nutritional foods, even if a mother gets birth, several children, she wouldn't be able to provide enough food during the gestation.

CONCLUSION

Bangladesh has been working to uplift and address maternal and child undermatron problems for years now. Consequently, Bangladesh has done well in MDGs concerning reduce child maternal deaths. But still, we cannot stall child and maternal death even ensuring adequate nutrition for all mothers and children are in a question. In this study, we have addressed some several factors which are responsible for childhood underweight in rural Bangladesh. The study connotes that there has much room to take off the situation otherwise rural children will continually be dying each year.

The more specific interventions need to be addressed concerning the aforesaid three intermediate objectives:

- To create a sustainable resilient food system for healthy diets which will be demonstrated through media partners and local governments as well as NGOs so that people from all levels follow.
- Effective plans and policies should be introduced to remove regional inequalities throughout the country.
- A social and nutrition-related education should be promoted from the grass-roots level of education.
- Along with national health systems for ensuring nutrition needs universally recognized nutritional interventions should be aligned with our own.
- To be building strong nutritional governance and need to enhance accountability and transparency at all levels of implementing any policies and programs regarding ameliorating the nutritional status of the mother and children must be enforced through regular monitoring.

REFERENCES

[1] de Onis, Mercedes. "Child growth and development." In *Nutrition and Health in a Developing World*, pp. 119-141. Humana Press, Cham, 2017.

[2] Rahman, Azizur and Soma Chowdhury. "Determinants of chronic malnutrition among preschool children in Bangladesh. *Journal of Biosocial Science*, *39*(2), (2007), 161-173. https://doi.org/10.1017/S0021932006001295.

[3] Mendez, Michelle A., and Linda S. Adair. "Severity and timing of stunting in the first two years of life affect performance on cognitive tests in late childhood." *The Journal of nutrition* 129, no. 8 (1999): 1555-1562.

[4] Pollitt, Ernesto, Kathleen S. Gorman, Patrice L. Engle, Reynaldo Martorell, Juan Rivera, Theodore D. Wachs, and Nevin S. Scrimshaw. "Early supplementary feeding and cognition: effects over two decades." *Monographs of the Society for Research in Child Development* (1993): i-118.

[5] World Health Organization. *Maternal anthropometry and pregnancy outcomes: a WHO collaborative study*. No. 73. World Health Organization, 1995.

[6] Martorell, Reynaldo. "Long-term consequences of growth retardation during early childhood." *Human growth: basic and clinical aspects* (1992): 143-149.

[7] Rahman, Azizur and Biswas, C. Soma. Nutritional status of under-5 children in Bangladesh. *South Asian Journal of Population and Health*, *2*(1), (2009), 1-11.

[8] Megabiaw, Berihun and Rahman, Azizur. Prevalence and determinants of chronic malnutrition among under-5 children in Ethiopia. *International Journal of Child Health and Nutrition*, *3*(2), (2013), 230-236. https://doi.org/10.6000/1929-4247.2013.02.03.5.

[9] Rahman, Azizur, Rahman, M. Sazedur and Rahman, M. Ashfikur. Determinants of infant mortality in Bangladesh: A nationally surveyed data analysis. *International Journal of Child Health and*

Nutrition, *8*(3), (2019), 93-102. https://doi.org/10.6000/1929-4247.2019.08.03.3.

[10] Rahman, Azizur, Chowdhury, Soma and Hossain, Delwar. Acute malnutrition in Bangladeshi children levels and determinants. *Asia-Pacific Journal of Public Health*, *21*(3), (2009), 294-302. https://doi.org/10.1177/1010539509335399.

[11] Rahman, Azizur and Sapkota, Mohesh. Knowledge on vitamin A rich foods among mothers of preschool children in Nepal: Impacts on public health and policy concerns. *Science Journal of Public Health*, *2*(4), (2014), 316-322. https://doi.org/10.11648/j.sjph.20140204.22.

[12] Black, Robert E., Lindsay H. Allen, Zulfiqar A. Bhutta, Laura E. Caulfield, Mercedes De Onis, Majid Ezzati, Colin Mathers, Juan Rivera, and Maternal and Child Undernutrition Study Group. "Maternal and child undernutrition: global and regional exposures and health consequences." *The lancet* 371, no. 9608 (2008): 243-260.

[13] de Onis, Mercedes, David Brown, Monika Blossner, and Elaine Borghi. *Levels and trends in child malnutrition. joint child malnutrition estimates*. Technical report, UNICEF Geneva and WHO Washington DC and World Bank, 2015. 1, 2015.

[14] Black, Robert E., Cesar G. Victora, Susan P. Walker, Zulfiqar A. Bhutta, Parul Christian, Mercedes De Onis, Majid Ezzati et al. "Maternal and child undernutrition and overweight in low-income and middle-income countries." *The Lancet* 382, no. 9890 (2013): 427-451.

[15] Das, Sumonkanti, Azizur Rahman, Ashraf Ahamed, and Sabbir T. Rahman. "Multi-level models can benefit from minimizing higher-order variations: An illustration using child malnutrition data." *Journal of Statistical Computation and Simulation 89*, no. 6 (2019): 1090-1110.

[16] Rahman, Azizur. "Estimating small area health-related characteristics of populations: A methodological review." *Geospatial Health 12*, no. 1 (2017): 3-14.

[17] Talukder, Ashis. "Factors associated with malnutrition among under-five children: illustration using Bangladesh demographic and health survey, 2014 data." *Children* 4, no. 10 (2017): 88.

[18] Aheto, Justice Moses K., Thomas J. Keegan, Benjamin M. Taylor, and Peter J. Diggle. "Childhood Malnutrition and Its Determinants among Under-Five Children in Ghana." *Paediatric and perinatal epidemiology* 29, no. 6 (2015): 552-561.

[19] Rahman, Azizur, Soma Chowdhury, Abdul Karim, and Sultan Ahmed. "Factors associated with nutritional status of children in Bangladesh: A multivariate analysis." *Demography India* 37, no. 1 (2008): 95-109.

[20] Nahar, Baitun, Tahmeed Ahmed, Kenneth H. Brown, and Md Iqbal Hossain. "Risk factors associated with severe underweight among young children reporting to a diarrhoea treatment facility in Bangladesh." *Journal of health, population, and nutrition* 28, no. 5 (2010): 476.

[21] Rahman, Azizur. "Significant risk factors for childhood malnutrition: evidence from an Asian developing country." *Science Journal of Public Health* 4, no. 1-1 (2016): 16-27.

[22] Rayhan, Md Israt, and M. Sekander Hayat Khan. "Factors causing malnutrition among under five children in Bangladesh." *Pak J Nutr* 5, no. 6 (2006): 558-62.

[23] Chowdhury, Mohammad Rocky Khan, Mohammad Shafiur Rahman, Mohammad Mubarak Hossain Khan, Mohammad Nazrul Islam Mondal, Mohammad Mosiur Rahman, and Baki Billah. "Risk factors for child malnutrition in Bangladesh: a multilevel analysis of a nationwide population-based survey." *The Journal of pediatrics* 172 (2016): 194-201.

[24] Pramod Singh, G. C., Manju Nair, Ruth B. Grubesic, and Frederick A. Connell. "Factors associated with underweight and stunting among children in rural Terai of eastern Nepal." *Asia Pacific Journal of Public Health* 21, no. 2 (2009): 144-152.

[25] Adhikari, Deepak, Resham Bahadur Khatri, Yuba Raj Paudel, and Amod Kumar Poudyal. "Factors associated with underweight among

under-five children in eastern Nepal: community-based cross-sectional study." *Frontiers in Public Health* 5 (2017): 350.

[26] *National Institute of Population Research and Training - NIPORT/Bangladesh, Mitra and Associates/Bangladesh, and ICF International. "Bangladesh Demographic and Health Survey 2014." Dhaka: NIPORT, Mitra and Associates, and ICF International (2016).*

[27] McDonald, Christine M., Ibironke Olofin, Seth Flaxman, Wafaie W. Fawzi, Donna Spiegelman, Laura E. Caulfield, Robert E. Black, Majid Ezzati, Goodarz Danaei, and Nutrition Impact Model Study. "The effect of multiple anthropometric deficits on child mortality: meta-analysis of individual data in 10 prospective studies from developing countries." *The American journal of clinical nutrition* 97, no. 4 (2013): 896-901.

[28] Rahman, Azizur, and Md Sazedur Rahman. "Rural-Urban Differentials of Childhood Malnutrition in Bangladesh." *International Journal of Child Health and Nutrition* 8, no. 1 (2019): 35-42.

[29] Hong, Rathavuth, James E. Banta, and Jose A. Betancourt. "Relationship between household wealth inequality and chronic childhood under-nutrition in Bangladesh." *International Journal for Equity in Health* 5, no. 1 (2006): 15.

[30] Sharma, Deepak, Sweta Shastri, and Pradeep Sharma. "Intrauterine growth restriction: antenatal and postnatal aspects." *Clinical Medicine Insights: Pediatrics* 10 (2016): CMPed-S40070.

[31] Ayana, Amsalu Bokore, Tsedeke Wolde Hailemariam, and Alemu Sufa Melke. "Determinants of acute malnutrition among children aged 6–59 months in Public Hospitals, Oromia region, West Ethiopia: a case–control study." *BMC Nutrition* 1, no. 1 (2015): 34.

[32] Rahman, Azizur, and Ann Harding. "Small area estimation and microsimulation modeling." Boca Raton, USA: CRC Press, 2017.

[33] Fentahun, Wagaye, Mamo Wubshet, and Amare Tariku. "Undernutrition and associated factors among children aged 6-59 months in East Belesa District, northwest Ethiopia: a community

based cross-sectional study." *BMC public health* 16, no. 1 (2016): 506.

[34] Negash, Canaan, Susan J. Whiting, Carol J. Henry, Tefera Belachew, and Tewodros G. Hailemariam. "Association between maternal and child nutritional status in Hula, rural Southern Ethiopia: A cross sectional study." *PloS one* 10, no. 11 (2015): e0142301.

[35] Bairagi, Radheshyam. "Is income the only constraint on child nutrition in rural Bangladesh?" *Bulletin of the World Health Organization* 58, no. 5 (1980): 767.

In: Malnutrition
Editor: Azizur Rahman
ISBN: 978-1-53617-597-4

Chapter 7

MITIGATE CHILD MALNUTRITION IN DEVELOPING COUNTRIES VIA KNOWLEDGE EXTRACTION TECHNIQUES

M. G. N. A. S. Fernando, PhD [*]***, Dinuni K. Fernando, PhD***[†]***,***
S. N. Ariyadasa[‡]***, L. K. Munasinghe***[§]
and S. H. D. Senanayake[¶]
Department of Information Systems Engineering,
University of Colombo School of Computing, Sri Lanka

Abstract

Child malnutrition is one of the major health concerns that affect the economic growth of a country as children are the future workforce. Further, child malnutrition critically impacts economic growth of a developing country than a developed country. Geographical conditions, poverty index, education level, food habits, cultural traditions may play significant role when deciding malnutrition. Further, country to country impact of these factors may vary. Considering current state of the art there is no such study investigate means of child malnutrition (age under 5 years) in Sri Lankan context. Main objective of this research is to establish an

[*]Corresponding Author's Email: nas@ucsc.cmb.ac.lk.
[†]Corresponding Author's Email: dkf@ucsc.cmb.ac.lk.
[‡]Corresponding Author's Email: ariyadasahmsn@gmail.com.
[§]Corresponding Author's Email: lkmunasinghe@gmail.com.
[¶]Corresponding Author's Email: senanayakeshd@gmail.com.

knowledge rich environment for related parties to make decisions to reduce child malnutrition condition in a developing country context (eg: Sri Lanka) by considering rule based data mining techniques. Our experimental results show that the education of the parents, access for media for the knowledge, proper understanding of family planning are crucial factors from preventing children falling into malnutrition condition. Further, results shows that "Tamil" ethnicity shows higher probability to malnourished due to food consumption pattern. Further, lack of nutrition during pregnancy impacts child health and malnutrition condition.

Keywords: child malnutrition, data mining, Sri Lankan malnutrition, classification

1. INTRODUCTION

Child malnutrition is one of the critical health indication that negatively impact the future economic growth of a country. Malnutrition is a broad term that commonly refers to under-nutrition. The under-nutrition build upon consisting three categories, namely, underweight, stunting and wasting. However, malnutrition also technically used to refer both under and over nutrition [6_def]. The term under-nourished refers when the diet does not provide adequate calories, protein and minerals to maintain the growth of a child. According to WHO Global Database [2] on Child Growth and Malnutrition claims that Sri Lanka shows 25.5% of underweight, 23.8% of stunting, 13.7% of wasting and 0.3% of overweight. Based on statistics, over-nutrition is not visible in Sri Lankan context compared to other countries. Therefore it is reasonable to consider child malnutrition as under-nutrition considering current Sri Lankan context. Further, one of the main cause of increment in child mortality is child malnutrition. WHO claims that nearly 50% child deaths are reported due to child malnutrition. According to Millennium Development Goals [3], child mortality is the fourth goal that need to be reduce for the betterment of a country. Therefore, by considering all these facts, finding a better solution for the economic development via advanced technology to reduce child malnutrition requires serious attention. Technologies such as data mining, statistical methods and machine learning techniques can be used to find an reliable solution to minimize the existence of child malnutrition in Sri Lankan context. Section 2 discusses research problem and section 3 discusses research objective of the proposing problem. Section 4 discuss current state of the art of child malnutrition and section 5 explore methodologies of our research. Section 6 gives the ndings of the research and section 7 brings up the discussion by mentioning the applicability of the knowledge in community perspective and finally section 7 gives the conclusion with future work of the research area.

2. Problem Statement

When comparing the literature based on the current state of the art, majority of studies related to malnutrition are based on statistical analysis. For every six years of time, Demography and Health Survey (DHS) is conducted most of the countries to capture individual and social background information. Considering existing literature, we had couple of questions related to the domain of child malnutrition. Were these data analyzed to nd hidden patterns? Whether the improved techniques such as data mining were used to solve the problem? Most of the times, answer is NO. Although several statistical based researches have been carried out in this area, are those enough to predict whether a child will affect the malnutrition in future? Still these are niche areas and most researchers have not address this issue. As we discussed above, child malnutrition makes a negative impact on future economic growth. According to the standards of World Health Organization (WHO), Sri Lanka is in very severe stage in child malnutrition. According to their claims, wasted, underweight and stunted children are the main cause for child malnutrition [2]. Child malnutrition shows linear relationship to child mortality rate. Further, achieving millennium development goals is another concern. Therefore, data modeling and analysis tools, such as data mining, have the potential to generate a knowledge-rich environment which can help to significantly improve the quality of decision marking in this major health factor. Throughout this research, the strength of this data mining is used to excavate hidden knowledge to build that environment, which ultimately helps our nation to place a big step in near future.

3. Research Objectives

Main objective of this research is to produce knowledge rich environment, which helps responsible parties to make decisions to reduce child malnutrition condition in Sri Lanka. Apart of the major objective, there are few other minor objectives as well. Namely, to support achieve millennium development goals, produce healthy future generation to support future economic growth of the country. The aim of this research is to nd solutions to three main research questions to achieve the above objectives. Main questions are, 1) what are the causes for child malnutrition?, 2) what are the impacts of this child malnutrition? and 3) how to minimize the prevalence of child malnutrition?. The rst two questions may provide better answers when considering existing literature and by examining Sri Lankan and other regional context. Third question can be analyzed by data sources.

4. Related Work

According to John Hopkins Medicine [4], Malnutrition is a condition that develops in the body when body is deprived of essential vitamins, minerals and other basic nutrients it needs to maintain healthy tissues and organ function. Several researches and cross-country studies have been carried out to combat child malnutrition in past. However, considering statistics [5], from 6.8 billion world population, 13.6% shows child malnutrition. Further, it shows, entirely undernourished percentage belongs to developing countries. According to UNICEF [6] statistics, South Asia has staggered high levels of underweight prevalence and among them 40% of them are under five in age. Despite, Sri Lanka belongs to south Asia, UNICEF claims that Bangladesh, India and Pakistan account for the half the world underweight children (i.e, 29% compared to developing world under 5 age population). Several studies have investigated child malnutrition in south Asian region [7] such as Bangladesh [8, 9, 10, 11], Nepal [12] and Africa [13]. Considering nutritional status of pre-school children in Sri Lanka, according to claims [14] of Department of Census and Statistics, overall 30% of children (under 5 age) are moderately or severely underweight and another 36% are found to be moderately underweight. Although Sri Lanka's malnutrition prevalence is lower compared to other South Asian regional countries, but it is in very severe stage compared to developed countries. Severity of malnutrition is further elaborated [15, 16] as follows. Sri Lanka has identified as a country that severe suffers underweight, stunted and wasted conditions in children less than 5 years of age. Further, it states that Child malnutrition in Sri Lanka is significantly high in numbers. Nearly one in three children in the age group 3-59 months is underweight, and more than 1 in 10 children in this age group suffers with chronic or acute malnutrition. Therefore we analyzed the existing literature under several domains mainly causes of malnutrition, impact and methodologies used to solve child malnutrition through various researches over different geographical boundaries.

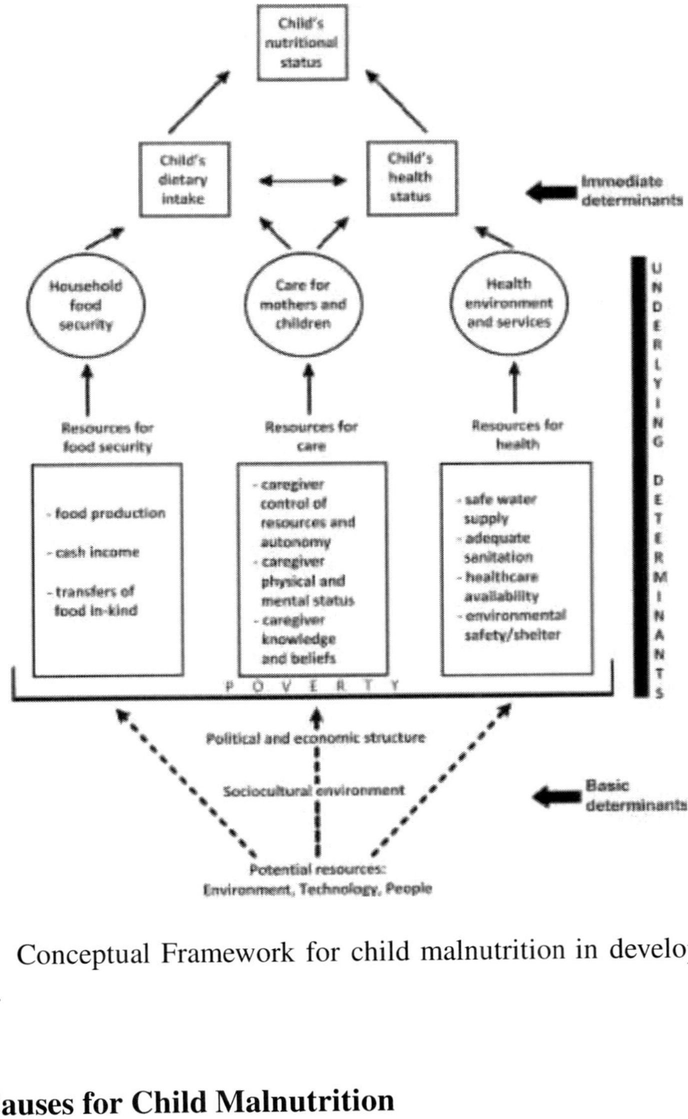

Figure 1. Conceptual Framework for child malnutrition in developing countries [17].

4.1. Causes for Child Malnutrition

Crucial factors that affecting malnutrition includes poverty, cost of food, dietary practices and agriculture productivity [18]. Smith et al. [17] proposes a conceptual framework (shown in Fig. _figurefig:smith_figure) that shows immediate and basic, underlying determinants of child malnutrition. According to the findings, dietary intake and the health status are considered to be the immediate causes. Food security like per capita national food availability, womens education and status related to mens and health environment quality such as safe water access are considered to be underlying causes. Chirstianensen et al. [19] proposes a similar study in the context of Ethiopia. According the findings, child care, sanitation availability, sewerage facilities, parental education, food cost and maternal education listed as key determinants of child nutrition. Further study elaborates that individual characteristics such as genetic endowment, gender, age, community characteristics (eg: distance to nearest health center, safe drinking water, flush toilet usage) relies on the nutrition production.

Per capita national income and political environment are basic determinants of country's economic growth that directly impacts child malnutrition. Study of Lian et al. [20] is based macro level data of families and the community. Identied factors are categorized as biological (i.e, age and birth weight), behavioral (i.e, weaning age, weaning duration, number of hospital admission, percentage of calorie/Reference Nutrient Intake (RNI), percentage of protein/RNI, frequency of receive treatment, mothers family planning and breastfeeding duration) or environmental aspect (i.e, total expenditure per month, number of rooms in the house, total household income and socioeconomic index).

Millennium Development Goals that were introduced by world bank [16] are directly related to Sri Lanka. Conceptual framework of Smith et al. [17] have included many of the related factors (i.e, age patterns, birth order and gender disparities, mothers age at birth) with high layer description. Although findings of Millennium Development Goals have considers Smith et al. conceptual framework however, their framework does not give a clear overview of these main factors. Further some researches discuss the key determinant causes as household resources like investment on child care, available sanitation and sewerage facilities; parental education, food prices, inequitable allocation of food among family members, income of mother, family size, number of children, birth order and maternal education knowledge affect childs nutritional stage. They further claim that the production of nutrition depends on set of inputs like, food, the utilization of health services, a series of exogenous individual characteristics like childs genetic endowment, gender and age; community characteristics like distance to the nearest health center, safe drinking water and ush toilets. However [19, 21] discuss that mothers diagnostic capabilities like childs nutrition and childs growth status also affects child malnutrition condition. Department of Census and Statistic in Sri Lanka claim that the nutritional status of a person depends on the quantity and quality of food available in the market, purchasing power of the household, the accessibility to food and the distribution of food within the household. In the case of children under five years of age, it depends on living standards, water and sanitation, birth weight, birth interval, parity, sex of child, weaning practices and mothers education. As per the analysis, dietary inadequacy is certainly the basic cause of malnutrition in pre-school children by National Demographic Health Survey in year 2000 [22].productive age group are malnourished and 17% of children under five years have been born as low birth weight babies. The illness, Diarrhea is also having a negative impact on child growth. Study revealed that 7% of children under five years of age, had suffered from at least one attack of diarrhea in the two weeks reference period. The prevalence rates are highest and stand at 13% for children in the (6-11) months age group, when solid food are introduced to the childs diet. The Income and Expenditure Survey [23] carried out in 2002 reveals that nearly one fourth (23.9%) of households in Sri Lanka falls into the category of poor household in terms of adequacy in energy intake [24]. According to these information it is justifiable that above mentioned factors have a clear impact on occurrence of malnutrition condition among Sri Lankan children. When comparing Smith's framework with Sastry's framework [25], Sastry introduces more factors considering family size, number of children, age and gender of children and birth order as key determinants than Smith. Therefore we believe that combining Smith's framework with Sastry can result a holistic framework for child malnutrition.

4.2. Consequences of Child Malnutrition

When a child gets infected by malnutrition there is a high probability of more disease infections to his or her body. Malnourished children are expected to have impaired immune systems, poorer cognitive development, and lower productivity at the adulthood and greater vulnerability to diet related chronic diseases such as hypertension coronary heart [17]. Factors such as mortality, morbidity, poor cognitive, motor development and less productivity can be some consequence malnutrition situation [26]. Further, [27] states that malnutrition significantly contributing for losses in Gross Domestic Product and also leads to more than 10% reduction of lifetime earnings per each malnourished individual, thus reduces GDP as well.

4.3. Methodologies Used

In section we discuss data gathering and analysis mechanisms that were used in existing literature. Kasirye et al. [28] have used a questionnaire for collecting data containing womens background characteristics, contraceptive usage details, their husbands background characteristics. The targeted children population was below the age of ve years. The clustering and stratication techniques were incorporated when deciding on the sample selection of the survey. The Z-score and regression methods were incorporated for analyzing the data. Rathnayake et al. [21]proposes commonly used measures for malnutrition are nutrient intake, calorie adequacy ratio and relative calorie allocation. Also authors claim protein energy malnutrition reasoning for anemia and goiter. Further they have reported nearly 14% of children in the age group of 3-59 months are stunted. The survey was carried out by a field gathered by a eld survey using a structured questionnaire in Sri Lankan limited to urban Kandy district. Dezhi et al. [24] proposed malnutrition condition in Sri Lanka considering rule based classification methods. Their developed system detects vulnerability to child malnutrition by considering rule combinations. Cheah et al. [20] have incorporated face-to-face interviews with questionnaires considering Sastry's conceptual framework. After the data collection statistical analysis was conducted. Based on the findings, authors claim that main factors that contribute to child malnutrition (age < 5 years) are total household income, total expenditure, number of rooms in the house and socio- economic status. Among these four factors, authors claim key determinant factor is socio-economic status.

Considering all proposed approach, Z-core approach is a main indication that used almost all researches to determine whether a child is malnourished or not. It is acceptable to use public international and cross country data standards like NCHS or CDC or WHO standards to find the Z-score values related to the children's height, weight and age. The literature has stated that if a child with the Z-score less than -3, he is severely malnourished. If the Z-score falls between -3 and -2, he is moderately malnourished. By the way, greater than -2 and less than 2 indicates that the child is in normal condition. By considering most of the related work, they are mostly limited to statistical approaches [29, 30], and very few have incorporated data mining techniques and very limited research focusing malnutrition in Sri Lankan context for under 5 age. Most existing approached are limited to small sample sizes. However, none of past work have consider existing publicly available cross country data from Department of Census in Sri Lanka. In our research we will be focusing on finding more features that can relate to child malnutrition for under age 5 for Sri Lankan context using data mining techniques.

5. Methodology

In our research, the knowledge discovery in databases (KDD) process in data mining was incorporated as the main methodology. The KDD process contains selection, preprocessing, transformation, data mining, evaluation and interpretation of data. In the selection stage, the children below ve years of age were selected. Next we handled missing elds and data inconsistencies via preprocessing stage. Data reduction and normalization techniques are used to formulate the nal data source during the transformation stage prior to mining stage. Then classication technique and decision tree mining model was used to handle the mining process.

Considering our data and objectives we identified that the association and classification technique are the best techniques and association rules and decision trees are the best data mining algorithms to be used for our model. Some key ndings were obtained by applying association and classification techniques over the data source. As the nal result of this KDD process, knowledge is illustrated through stage of interpretation.

5.1. Data Source

The Demography and Health Survey (DHS) 2006/2007 data set from Department of Census and Statistics [14] was used as the primary data source. Initially, the data source contained 25 tables and most of the tables contained over 80000 records. This DHS data source was used as training and testing data sets as the research was followed the supervised learning method. The attribute Malnourished is identified as the predictable attribute with value Y for children who have malnutrition and value N for children who havent malnutrition in current context. The attribute id was used as the key to nd specific child; the rest are input attributes.

5.2. Statistical Analysis

As the initial step, statistical analysis was carried according to the predictable attribute. Based on the data source, child malnutrition percentage was 34.86% and numbers were comparably similar to the recent past [31].

Since research followed the WHO standards and few literature was shown that some considerable increment was there under stunted and wasted children category in 2007 based on the past DHS data [31], 34.86% was accepted. Through the analysis, children in 2 year of age were suffering highly with this condition. Then, Eastern province had a lot of affected children and nearly 50% of state sector children were being contributed for this present condition. Religion wise, Hindu was contributed by 50%. In gender, there was no any signicant difference between male and female. Both were contributed by 35%. Further analysis were shown that the children who were not accessing safe food, media, iodized salt, etc and who were affected by Tsunami had been contributed to present situation. Also in the childrens house, when the number of rooms were being increased, the contribution was decreased. The data source was elaborated that the condition was nearly 40% for 2 rooms and when 6 or more, then the contribution was fallen down into 25%. House ownership also may be a matter for this condition and statistics was shown that 40% contribution from families who had not house ownerships and 34% from opposite. Further analysis was shown that families who had and had not farm houses were contributed by 34% and 39% respectively. In the analysis an abnormal behavior was found related to the fathers residence. Data source was shown that malnutrition condition was 35% when the father was there and 24% when he was not. Another one was the number of children for a same mother. Here when the number of children were being increased, contribution to the condition was also increased. Families with 5 or more children were contributed by 50% and with 2 were only 30%. Other attributes had been shown some general behavior with the predictable attribute and with the acquired knowledge within this phase was guided the research in to next stage, which was the KDD process.

5.3. Data Selection

As the initial step of data collection, age 5 years or less children group was filtered from the completed DHS data set. Filtered data with aged less than 5 year ended up to 6996 records. The selected data set comprised of general data (e.g., age, weight, height, etc.), household data (e.g., sanitation facilities, sewerage facilities, household conditions, etc.), and data of parents (e.g., parental education, alcoholism, etc.) per each child. The domain knowledge gathered through the literature was used for that selection process.

5.4. Data Processing

In pre-processing stage, rst data inconsistencies were. For example, data source consist of child's date of birth, however, mentioned date of birth may denoted as the interviewed day for some data records. Some data records shows repeated data e.g., date of birth by the interviewer. Therefore such inconsistencies were removed by mapping two records. Missing values of the data records were filled by considering Kamber et al. techniques [32]. For filling missing values we considered techniques namely 1) ignore the tuple, 2) ll in the missing value manually, 3) the attribute mean to ll in the missing value, and 4) the most probable value to ll in the missing value. After handling inconsistencies, missing values and duplicates data source was transferred to the transformation process.

5.5. Data Transformation

The preprocessed data requires some sort of transformation; to be able to apply particular data mining algorithms. Data reduction techniques such as dimension reduction and feature selection methods, normalization methods were used in this transformation stage. The Z-score normalization process was used to categorize the children to check whether they are malnourished or not. The attributes which had much variation of categorical values were reduced to manageable amount of categories. After that data cleaning process, the data source was reduced to 6714 records. These cleaned data could be feed into mining model to produce hidden patterns and relationships.

5.6. Data Mining

After completing the above stages, data source is ready for the mining purposes. Prior to mining, data source is divided into two sets, namely training and test data sets. Then mining models are applied to the training data set to learn patterns and relationships. Decision tree was the mining model that we used in this stage. J48 algorithm in WEKA1 was the supporting software used to make the data mining process easy. The selected classifier was J48 and the predictable attribute was the leaf node attribute. Then WEKA application generated the decision tree for the provided data source. By using several combinations of attributes with predictable attribute, we ended up with few decision trees that were incorporated to make rules. The rules with the probability of 75% or higher were considered with the predictable attribute value Y. 19 rules were identified from generated decision trees.

6. RESULTS

After narrowing down the rules through mining model, next task was to evaluate the rules.The test data set was selected to evaluate the 19 rules. Then we only selected the rules with 75% or more in the test data source that nally ended up with 7 rules. Seven final rules are mentioned below.

1. Ethnicity = T AND Single Birth = N ⇒ Malnourished (83.33%)
2. M Schooling = N AND F Alive = Y AND Living Same House = Y AND Pregnant Now = N AND M Suffering Disease = N AND M Rubella Vaccine = Y AND Total Child Birth = 4 AND Birth Expected Time = N ⇒ Malnourished (100%)
3. M Schooling = N AND F Alive = Y AND Living Same House = Y AND Pregnant Now = N AND M Suffering Disease = N AND M Rubella Vaccine = N AND Contraceptive Used = Y AND Total Child Birth = 5M ⇒ Malnourished (100%)
4. Bank Access = Y AND Iodized Salts = Y AND Mosquito Protected = N AND Tsunami Affected = N AND Agriculture Land = Y AND Media Access = N AND House Owner = N ⇒ Malnourished (100%)
5. Bank Access = Y AND Iodized Salts = N AND Farm Animal = N AND Agriculture Land = Y AND Mosquito Protected = N ⇒ Malnourished (75%)
6. M Schooling = Y AND Bank Access = N AND Single Birth = Y AND Tsunami Affected = N AND Safe Water Access = Y AND Iodized Salts = Y AND Mosquito Protected = Y AND Only Breast Fed Duration = 4M6M AND Cesarean Delivery = Y AND Ethnicity = T ⇒ Malnourished (75%)

7. M Schooling = Y AND Bank Access = N AND Single Birth = N $\Rightarrow$ Malnourished (86.36%)

7. DISCUSSION

From the results, it shows that the education of the parents, access for media for the knowledge, proper understanding of family planning are crucial factors from preventing children falling into malnutrition condition. It is evident that there is a high probability for children belongs to "Tamil" ethnicity to be malnourished. This observation can be justied by the food consumption patterns of them as most them consume vegetarian foods with an unbalanced diet. They may not get the sufficient amount of nutrients to cope with malnutrition condition. Also the distribution of the Tamil population is quite high in estate sector (which is known as less developed and poverty striking region in most of the cases.) When the number of children grows in a family, parents may not have the ability to give their children the required nutrients sufficiently due to their financial status. This may be the reason for the high probability of malnutrition occurrence in children who are from the families who are having more than three children. The result also implies that the occurrence of malnutrition is high for children those who were born as twins. The reasons for this may be the mothers do not get required nutrients sufficiently during their pregnancy and after birth it is hard to maintain two or more children at the same time with sufficient care. If a child conceived in a time period that the parents did not expect, the child may not get the required care from the parents. This must be the reason behind such children having a high probability of getting caught by child malnutrition. There is a belief in the society that if a childs parents are there with them the probability of child being malnourished is significantly low. But as per the ndings we can see that the child can be a victim of child malnutrition even if it is true; depending on a combination of other factors as discussed above. The results indicate that the children from agricultural based families can also be malnourished. That may be due to those families are inclined to adhere to same kind of food they grow, without reaching for a variation of food types for a balanced diet and also they might not getting an enough income from their occupation to go for more variation.

Conclusion

The child malnutrition is a significant factor that decrements countrys economic growth. We have incorporated data mining approach to uncover relationships which leads to ways and means for child malnutrition. Key factors that affects child malnutrition obtained from the research were lack of parent education, lack of media access, insufficient knowledge of family planning and family wealth. Health domain experts can contribute to established biological background for these findings from our research. Generated knowledge can be used by the responsible parties to come up new strategies to further reduce child malnutrition condition. Further, similar methodology can be applied to developing countries to reduce child malnutrition conditions.

Future work includes, automating the data feeding process for a task oriented data mart with several years of DHS data. Aiming for generating knowledge on child malnutrition. Using that knowledge of several years the country will be able to predict the condition in future years and get the appropriate actions and preventative measures. Incorporating genetic endowment to add the same methodology which might lead to more interesting results.

References

[1] *UNICEF*. malnutrition denition popup.https://www.unicef.org/ progressforchildren/2006n4/malnutritiondefinition.html, 2006 (accessed November, 2019).

[2] *WHO*. who—sri lanka. http://www.who.int/nutgrowthdb/database/ countries/lka/en/, 2017.

[3] United Nations. *Millennium development goals*. http://www.who.int/ nutgrowthdb/database/countries/lka/en/, 2015.

[4] John Hopkins Medicine. *What is malnutrition?* https://www.hopkinsmedicine.org/ health/conditions-and-diseases/ malnutrition.

[5] World Hunger Educational Service. *2011 world hunger and poverty facts and statistics*. http://www.worldhunger.org/articles/Learn/world.html.

[6] UNICEF. *1 in 2: Approximately 1 in 2 underweight children in the developing world live in South Asia.* https://www.unicef.org/ factoftheweek/index_49638.html .

[7] Rahman Azizur. Significant risk factors for childhood malnutrition: Evidence from an asian developing country. *Science Journal of Public Health*, 4:16–27, 01 2016.

[8] Rahman Azizur and Biswas Soma. Determinants of chronic malnutrition among preschool children in bangladesh. *Journal of biosocial science*, 39:161–73, 04 2007.

[9] Rahman Azizur. Geospatial, socioeconomic, demographic and health determinants of childhood mortality in bangladesh. *Demography India: population - society - economy - environment - interactions*, 48(2):74–85, 2019.

[10] Rahman Azizur and Rahman Md. Rural-urban differentials of childhood malnutrition in bangladesh. *International Journal of Child Health and Nutrition*, 8:35–42, 03 2019.

[11] Rahman Azizur, Chowdhury Soma, and Hossain Delwar. Acute malnutrition in bangladeshi children: Levels and determinants. *Asia Pacific Journal of Public Health*, 21(3):294–302, 2009.

[12] Rahman Azizur and Sapkota Mahesh. Knowledge on vitamin a rich foods among mothers of preschool children in nepal: Impacts on public health and policy concerns. *Science Journal of Public Health*, 2:316, 01 2014.

[13] Zeleke Berihun and Rahman Azizur. Prevalence and determinants of chronic malnutrition among under-5 children in ethiopia. *International Journal of Child Health and Nutrition*, 2:230–236, 08 2013.

[14] Department of Census and Statistics of Sri Lanka. *Nutritional status of pre-school children in Sri Lanka.* http://www.statistics.gov.lk/social/nutrition%20status.pdf .

[15] Chhabra Ritu and Rokx Claudia. *The nutrition mdg indicator: Interpreting progress*, 2004.

[16] World Bank. *Millennium development goals of Sri Lanka: Child malnutrition.* http://www.worldhunger.org/articles/Learn/world.html.

[17] Smith Lisa C. and Haddad Lawrence. *Explaining child malnutrition in developing countries: A cross-country analysis*, 1999.

[18] Tette Edem M. A., Sifah Eric K., and Nartey Edmund T. Factors affecting malnutrition in children and the uptake of interventions to prevent the condition. *BMC pediatrics*, 15:189, 2015.

[19] Christiaensen Luc and Alderman Harold. Child malnutrition in ethiopia: Can maternal knowledge augment the role of income? *Economic Development and Cultural Change*, 52:287–312, 02 2004.

[20] Lian Cheah Whye, Manan Wan, and Hussin Zabidi. A structural equation model of the determinants of malnutrition among children in rural kelantan, malaysia. *Rural and remote health*, 10:1248, 01 2010.

[21] Rathnayake Ishara and Weerahewa Jeevika. An assessment of intra-household allocation of food: A case study of the urban poor in kandy. *Sri Lankan Journal of Agricultural Economics*, 4, 08 2011.

[22] Department of Census and Statistics Sri Lanka. *Sri lanka - demographic and health survey - 2000.* http://nada.statistics.gov.lk/ index.php/catalog/1109 .

[23] Department of Census and Statistics Sri Lanka. *Household income and expenditure survey 2002.* http://www.statistics.gov.lk/HIES/HIES2002/InEx2002.pdf .

[24] Xu Dezhi and Ganegoda Upeksha. Rule based classification to detect malnutrition in children. *International Journal on Computer Science and Engineering*, 3, 01 2011.

[25] Sastry Narayan. Community characteristics, individual and household attributes, and child survival in brazil. *Demography*, 33(2):211,229, 1996-05.

[26] Gragnolati Michele, Shekar Meera, Gupta Monica Das, Bredenkamp Caryn, Lee Yi kyoung Gragnolati, Michele, Shekar Meera. Indias undernourished children: A call for reform and action. In *Health, Nutrition*

and Population (HNP). Discussion Paper. Washington D.C.: The World Bank, 2005.

[27] The Poverty Portal. *An information resource portal on poverty in Sri Lanka*. http://www.poverty portal.lk/blogs/blog-1-22.html.

[28] Kasirye Ibrahim. What are the successful strategies for reducing malnutrition among young children in east africa? *Human Development Report Office (HDRO), United Nations Development Programme (UNDP), Human Development Research Papers (2009 to present)*, 01 2010.

[29] Das Sumonkanti, Rahman Azizur, Ahamed Ashraf, and Rahman Sabbir Tahmidur. Multi-level models can benefit from minimizing higher-order variations: an illustration using child malnutrition data. *Journal of Statistical Computation and Simulation*, 89(6):1090–1110, 2019.

[30] Rahman Azizur, Chaudhury S., Karim Abdul, and Ahmed Sultan. Factors associated with nutritional status of children in bangladesh: A multivariate analysis. *Demography India*, 37:95–109, 07 2008.

[31] World Bank. *Malnutrition in Sri Lanka: Scale, scope, causes, and potential response*. https://openknowledge.worldbank.org/handle/10986/7656 , 2007.

[32] Han Jiawei and Kamber Micheline. *Data mining: Concepts and techniques*, 2000.

ABOUT THE EDITOR

Associate Professor Azizur Rahman, PhD
Charles Sturt University, Computing and Mathematics,
Wagga Wagga, New South Wales, Australia
Email: azrahman@csu.edu.au

Associate Professor Azizur Rahman, PhD, is an applied statistician and data scientist with expertise in both developing and applying novel methodologies, models and technologies. He is the Leader of "Statistics and Data Mining Research Group" within the Data Science Research Unit at the Faculty of Business, Justice and Behavioural Sciences, Charles Sturt University (CSU). Prof. Rahman is able to assist in understanding multi-disciplinary research issues within various fields including how to understand the individual activities which occur within very complex behavioral, socio-economic and ecological systems.

He develops "alternative methods in microsimulation modelling technologies" which are very useful tools to socioeconomic policy analysis and evaluation. His 2016 book has contributed significantly to the field of small area estimation and microsimulation modelling. Prof. Rahman's research interests encompass issues in simple to multi-facet analyses in various fields ranging from the mathematical sciences to the law and legal studies. He has more than 100 scholarly publications including a few books. Prof. Rahman's research is funded by the Australian Federal and State Governments, and he serves on a range of editorial boards including the *International Journal of Microsimulation (IJM).* He obtained the SOCM Research Excellence Award 2018 and the CSU-RED Achievement Award 2019.

INDEX

M

N

O

P

V

W

Y

Z